Typhoid Fever

Typhoid Fever

A History

Richard Adler *and* Elise Mara

McFarland & Company, Inc., Publishers
Jefferson, North Carolina

LIBRARY OF CONGRESS CATALOGUING-IN-PUBLICATION DATA

Names: Adler, Rich, author. | Mara, Elise, 1992– author.
Title: Typhoid fever : a history / Richard Adler and Elise Mara.
Description: Jefferson, North Carolina : McFarland & Company, Inc.,
    Publishers, 2016. | Includes bibliographical references and index.
Identifiers: LCCN 2016001631 | ISBN 9780786497812 (softcover :
    acid free paper) ∞
Subjects: LCSH: Typhoid fever—History.
Classification: LCC RA644.T8 A35 2016 | DDC 616.9/272—dc23
LC record available at http://lccn.loc.gov/2016001631

BRITISH LIBRARY CATALOGUING DATA ARE AVAILABLE

ISBN (print) 978-0-7864-9781-2
ISBN (ebook) 978-1-4766-2209-5

Front cover: Richard Pfeiffer (standing) and Robert Koch (image
courtesy Wellcome Library, London)

Printed in the United States of America

*McFarland & Company, Inc., Publishers
    Box 611, Jefferson, North Carolina 28640
    www.mcfarlandpub.com*

Table of Contents

Acknowledgments

We would like to thank the following individuals for their support, monetarily and otherwise, in the writing of this book: John Cristiano and the Office of Sponsored Research at the University of Michigan–Dearborn; Doug Atkins of the National Institutes of Health, National Library of Medicine, for the extra, extra (intentionally repeated) effort he carried out in tracing copyrights; Rose Adler in helping prepare images; Jeff and Sue Mara for generally being supportive and encouraging one of us (E.M.) to continue working on this book; Sally Adler for her supportive help; and Rodney Foster, RN, who provided an appreciation and interest in epidemiology and for the human stories in public health.

Preface

> There is a fascination, a dramatic interest, in working out, even in imagination, the dark and devious paths and bypaths along which the microscopic parasites that afflict the human race travel to their appointed victims. Only the epidemiologist realizes the full meaning of the phrase, "the pestilence that walketh in darkness."—George Chandler Whipple[1]

Typhoid fever is a disease with a muddled past. It is likely that it—as well as other gastrointestinal illnesses—has been with us since antiquity. However, tracking it through the history of civilization is complicated by the fact that until the 19th century it remained difficult to reliably distinguish this illness from other fevers that had similar characteristics. Lacking the distinctive symptomology of infectious diseases such as smallpox or syphilis as it was first described in the 16th century, typhoid was frequently confused with typhus or malaria (indeed, typho-malaria was considered a specific illness well into the 19th century) in the years before advances in pathology and germ theory would shed light on the characteristics and etiology of the disease. This era of "loose" definitions survives even in the name itself: "typhoid," the "oid" referring to an organism believed distinct from others for which it may have been mistaken. Generally applied, the term was an adjective which literally meant "resembling typhus," the designation of typhus referring to the unpleasant odors emanating from putrefying material that were believed to be associated with, if not the direct cause of, disease. Other examples include the original applications of names which evolved into influenza or malaria.[2] "Typhoid" as the term was routinely used was thus less a discrete illness than a descriptor for a certain set of symptoms, a term applied inconsistently across a range of disorders. The terminology has also created confusion when crossing national boundaries. For example, the word *tyfus* referred to the designation of typhoid fever by the British. In German, the term was *fleckfieber*, or spotted fever, referring to the rash. In the United States, spotted fever refers to a tick-borne disease originally found in the Rocky Mountains.[3]

It is perhaps understandable that ancient physicians and historians had difficulty differentiating between the major "fevers": malaria, typhus and typhoid. Each of them exhibits very similar symptoms. Any attempt by modern historians to identify or diagnose such illnesses produces the challenge of not only dealing with what were largely observations—bodies warm to the touch or undefined blisters or rashes—but also in translating ancient terminology. Typhus and typhoid fever were particularly difficult to differentiate, as each could be characterized by a high, prolonged fever, the level of which could not be determined by the ancients, as well as headache, rash and abdominal pain. At least malaria, which unquestionably existed within the swamps and standing waters or any other place infested by mosquitoes, produced an intermittent or repetitive fever interspersed with chills—most of the time. Malaria was likely among the tertian (two-day interval) or quartan (three-day interval) fevers described by Hippocrates on this basis (see Chapter 2). The Roman historian and physician Aulus Cornelius Celsus (ca. 25 BCE–50 CE) provided almost a modern textbook description of malaria in his surviving text *De Medicina*:

> But quartans are simpler. The fevers begin with shivering, then a heat erupts, and then, the fever having ended, the next two days are free of it. On the fourth day it returns.
> However, tertian fevers surely have two types. The one type beginning and ending in the same manner as a quartan, the other with only this difference; that it allows one day to be free of it, and returns on the third. The other type is far more insidious, for it always returns on the third day, and out of forty-eight hours, thirty-six of them (although sometimes less or more) are occupied by the paroxysm. Neither does it completely halt during remission, but only takes a lighter course. This type most physicians call semitertian (intermittent with characteristics of both daily and tertian).[4]

Celsus was therefore able to differentiate the (intermittent) fever characteristic of malaria with that of typhoid or typhus.

It would require the scientific observations of physicians in both Europe and the United States during the middle and late 19th century to unravel the puzzle of what typhoid fever actually was and, equally important in the understanding of its etiology, what it was not. As was the situation with several of the significant gastrointestinal illnesses intensively studied during that century, such as cholera or dysentery, the isolation and identification of the agent came decades after its method of transmission—through sewage-contaminated water—was determined. One can make the argument that understanding the method of transmission and identifying the agent led directly to the establishment of public health departments in an increasing number of cities, both in Europe and the United States. The difficulty in isolating and identifying the typhoid bacillus, now placed within the genus *Salmonella*, led to the use of a surrogate marker, once known as *Bacterium coli* (now *Escherichia coli*), to identify water supplies contaminated with sewage. Generations of microbiology students have since been challenged with learning and understanding the methodology of numerous biochemical tests used in differentiating common soil microorganisms from those which signify potential problems.

So what, one may wonder, made it so difficult to discover the underlying cause of the disease? The challenge in identifying the actual etiological agent was understandable only in the context of 19th-century bacteriology. The typhoid agent is not a virus. In fact, it is not even a particularly unusual bacterium. *Salmonella* will grow on most of the standard laboratory media, whether in those of more modern times or in the extant media of the 19th century. Even Victor Vaughan, dean of the University of Michigan Medical School between 1891 and 1921 and among the most important of the bacteriologists during that era, acknowledged as much.[5] The problem, of course, required first the observation and isolation of the organism from the victim, and then linking the isolate with a specific disease. A few similar examples linking an agent with an infectious disease could be found through much of the latter half of the 19th century. Anthrax is one such case in point. But it was the institution of what became known as Koch's Postulates during the 1880s which provided a working guide to physicians attempting to identify an etiological agent. The eponymously named postulates, generally attributed to the German physician Robert Koch while often ignoring the earlier models on which the postulates were based, are relatively simple in their concept: (1) the agent should be present in all cases of the disease, while (usually) not present in the absence of the disease; (2) the agent should be grown in pure culture and following inoculation into a test animal; (3) should produce the same disease; and finally, (4) the same agent should be reisolated from the test animal. It was not until the latter years of that century that this could all be put in place for the more common bacterial diseases. But even after these concepts had been applied by Koch and his associates and the concepts had gained widespread acceptance, certain bacterial diseases failed to fall neatly within the principles of the postulates. For example, neither the comma bacillus of cholera nor Eberth's bacillus, as the typhoid agent was sometimes termed, produced their respective diseases in common laboratory animals. As a result, even Vaughan remained skeptical for a time of the alleged role played by Eberth's bacillus as the etiological agent of typhoid.

Even if the etiological agent was not immediately identified, the solution to prevention of not only typhoid but also to gastrointestinal diseases in general, should have been obvious, at least to our modern way of thinking: the proper disposal of sewage. Typhoid outbreaks have historically been associated with two features of civilization: (1) urban areas outgrowing their sources of clean water, and (2) the movement of armies. The two were often linked with each other. While ancient writings describe localized outbreaks[6] which might very well have been those of typhoid fever, the first clearly documented epidemic of what appears almost certainly to be typhoid was that of the so-called Plague of Athens.[7] Not surprisingly, the plague took place against the background of the Peloponnesian War between Athens and Sparta. As will be described in greater detail later, DNA recently extracted from the teeth of victims of the plague hastily buried in mass graves 2500 years ago was identified as that of the typhoid agent. Alexander the Great a century later may have likewise succumbed to typhoid while returning to the Middle East after conquering most of the known world. Typhoid outbreaks were hardly confined to the movement of ancient armies. During the Crimean War (1853–1856) over 16,000 British soldiers died. "Only" 2600 died directly from battle wounds, the remainder succumbing to disease, much of which was typhoid resulting from the abysmal handling of human waste. And lest we attribute such outbreaks to foreign "ignorance," during the Spanish-American War (1898) some 20 percent of American soldiers camped in the South suffered from the same disease. The source of the outbreak was readily identified: the lack of proper disposal of sewage which resulted in human waste contaminating the water supply.

Clarification of the historical uncertainty in the diagnosis of the disease as one which was distinct from other enteric fevers began in the 17th century. While carrying out autopsies, pathologists described an unusual feature in the intestines of some victims. The Peyer's patches, nodules which make up a portion of the local immune system, often appeared ulcerated.[8] The British physician Thomas Willis, during the 1650s, likewise observed this feature in patients who had succumbed to what was often referred to as "putrid fever." In his clinical description of the disease, Willis established the distinction between typhoid and certain other fevers with similar symptoms and was considered to be the first physician to do so.[9] Other physicians reported similar pathologies, including actual perforations in the intestine, but these were treated more as curiosities than as hallmarks of a specific disease. Obviously, ulceration was only observable during autopsy, so while the patient was alive there were few means to distinguish between the various diseases which produced similar fevers.

This did not stop physicians from trying, and some of them appear to have come close to distinguishing typhoid fever from other illnesses. In his 1737 *Essay on Fevers*, John Huxam referred to "putrid typhus" and "slow nervous fever," with the latter corresponding to typhoid's gradual and sustained characteristic fever.[10] Lacking solid evidence, Huxam's designations did not replace the varieties of categories and names that populated the early 18th century scientific literature, including such vague descriptions as "nervous fever," "brain fever," and "low fever." The term typhoid fever was among those which sometimes appeared; actual credit for popularizing the name is generally given to French pathologist Pierre-Charles-Alexandre Louis, who undertook his own examinations of Peyer's patches in the 1820s.[11]

The modern understanding of the disease, even though the etiological agent had yet to be identified, really began in the 1830s. Like much of the progress in medicine during that era, that knowledge first occurred largely in Europe. In part, this was the result of the increased industrialization taking place there at this time. Cities were beginning to grow at an unprecedented pace, and the populations were quickly exceeding the capacity of sewer systems to handle the "flow." Gastrointestinal diseases such as cholera—which first appeared in significant numbers in portions of Europe and England in the 1820s—and typhoid evolved into increasingly serious health problems for the masses. The aforementioned Frenchman Louis, and William Gerhard, one of his many students, determined that the damage observed in the Peyer's patches was associated with a specific fever. Though there was some resemblance to typhus—an entirely unrelated disease but one with some similarity in symptoms—the intestinal perforations typical of typhoid were not observed in regions in which typhus was present; the conclusion was that these had to be unique diseases.

By the latter years of the 19th century it was increasingly apparent that typhoid had some connection with sewage. The germ theory of disease ultimately provided the explanation. Typhoid fever had its origin in "the dejections of the bowels [which] probably contain the active germs in largest amount."[12] Still, the time delay between when a person might have been exposed—the incubation period—and when symptoms actually developed led to a number of odd interpretations as physicians attempted to reconcile the germ theory with the extant ideas of miasmas released from rotting sewage. In attempting to resolve the two competing theories, some believed the putrefaction process was necessary to release such poisons into the air. In order to prevent the formation of such miasmas, they thought feces must be disinfected as soon as it left the patient's body. While the miasmatic theory may have been incorrect, the principles of disinfection it promoted were sound.

The isolation and identification of the actual etiological agent during the 1880s created additional drama as scientists argued over the question of priority. As discussed later in this book, Karl Eberth, Edwin Klebs and Georg Gaffky each had a legitimate claim to the identification of the typhoid bacillus; each faced the challenges of attempting to apply Koch's postulates in confirming that identity. Regardless of whom should be given priority for that discovery, the identification of the etiological agent quickly led to a mechanism for diagnosis. Even here an argument developed on the question of priority: Georges-Fernand-Isidor Widal or Albert Grünbaum. Widal, now considered the developer of the eponymously named Widal test, followed up the work of Richard Pfeiffer who had demonstrated that serum obtained from a patient with typhoid, when mixed with the typhoid bacillus, would cause the bacteria to agglutinate. Widal's streamlining of the reaction in 1896 was adopted by health departments as a diagnostic tool and continues to be applied even 120 years later. The first vaccine effective in immunizing a person against typhoid was developed by the British physician Almroth Wright about the same time as the Widal test was developed. While the vaccine was available for the immunization of British troops during the Boer War in southern Africa (1899–1902), problems in supply and the historic difficulties in preventing fecal

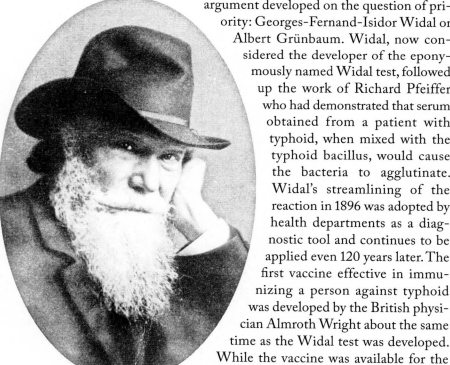

Karl Eberth (1835–1926), German bacteriologist credited with identifying the typhoid agent (courtesy National Library of Medicine).

contamination of water supplies—almost an occupational hazard in serving with the British army during the 19th century—resulted in widespread outbreaks of the disease among the troops. Of the approximately 550,000 men who served in the Boer campaign, an estimated 58,000 developed typhoid, with some 8,200 deaths, a number which exceeded the number of fatalities due to war wounds.[13] By comparison, the United States Army adopted Wright's vaccine in 1909, and unlike the situation in 1898 typhoid was not among the infectious disease problems encountered by the army during World War I (see Chapter 10).

The combination of vaccine development, the discovery of antibiotics, the development of treatments for water supplies—particularly the use of chlorine as a disinfectant—and, most important of all, the proper disposal of sewage have largely eliminated typhoid fever in the more economically developed countries. Still, it remains even today a significant health challenge in portions of the third world; as one example, an outbreak in central Africa in 2004 resulted in over 42,000 cases.

This book is the story of that disease, its possible presence in early civilizations and its impact on societies through the centuries. And while other sources describe the disease, few provide more than "lip service" to those individuals, many of whom are obscure figures in the history of medicine, whose work led to the understanding of the importance of proper sanitation and sewage disposal in the prevention of typhoid. We have attempted to highlight some of the more (and perhaps even less) significant individuals in that history. In this regard, we have researched what have often been overlooked bits of trifles. An example is found in Chapter 9 in the portion providing the history of "Typhoid Mary." Several accounts describe the first death attributed to Mary as the "lovely daughter" of William Bowen. We were unable to locate the young woman's name in these accounts. Death records available from the city of New York provided a (likely) name. While this may be of little use, or interest, to the historian, it was assuredly important to the family in 1907.

With the exception of an early chapter addressing the nature of the etiological agent itself, *Salmonella*, the story is largely chronological. It begins with the recounting of what are two of the arguably most famous outbreaks in the recorded history of typhoid: the Plague of Athens, already referred to briefly above, and the final illness and death of one of the most important figures in human history, Alexander the Great. Later chapters describe the deaths from typhoid fever of major figures from modern history, including Albert, Prince Consort and husband of Queen Victoria of Great Britain, and at least one (perhaps two) president of the United States.

However, much of the story takes place during the eighteenth and nineteenth centuries, when the first extensive description of what we now recognize as typhoid was reported by the English physician Thomas Willis, and when typhoid fever was subsequently established as a unique disease by the American physician William Wood Gerhard in the first half of the nineteenth century. Central to much of this work was the French physician and pathologist Pierre-Charles-Alexandre Louis, referred to briefly above, with whom Gerhard, and many others, studied. Their professional, and in some instances, personal, lives provide a human element to the developing research of the illness. As we shall see, one could artificially divide the understanding of typhoid into the "pre–Louis" era and the "post–Louis" era.

We also include some anecdotes and trivia to lighten up the story. We can begin with the seemingly simple question of the genus name of the etiological agent for typhoid fever: *Salmonella*, named for Daniel Elmer Salmon (1850–1914). The student of trivia might pose the question of why. Salmon did not discover the typhoid agent; in fact he was not even the individual who first isolated *Salmonella* from an infected animal. There are no shortages of clichés here, not least of which might be "rank has its privileges."

The story is an example of how mistaken interpretations of a scientific discovery potentially provide the scientist with unexpected answers to other problems. Hog cholera, sometimes referred to as swine fever, was, and in much of the world remains, a highly contagious often fatal infection of not only swine but also other animals. Similar viruses also are the etiological agents of disease in cattle and sheep. During the 1880s the United States Department of Agriculture had been carrying out systematic attempts to isolate and identify the etiological agent of the disease. The pathologist Theobald Smith (1859–1934), a newly hired addition to the Bureau of Animal Industry, a branch within the department, isolated from the abdomen and other tissues of infected animals a bacterium which he believed to be the etiological agent. Since Smith's director was Daniel Salmon, the new isolate was given the genus name *Salmonella* despite the fact Salmon had not been the specific scientist responsible for its isolation. Since the bacterium was thought to be the agent of hog cholera, its official name was designated as *Salmonella cholerae-suis*.[14,15] It was only in 1978 that the actual etiological agent of hog cholera, an RNA virus in the Flavivirus group, was correctly identified.[16]

The challenges which Smith faced in identifying the correct agent were twofold. First, the actual agent was a virus, the biological concept of which was unknown in the 1880s. (It should be pointed out here that the term virus was frequently used in the 19th century to designate an infectious agent such as a bacterium, and not the physical entity we think of today.) Equally important, recognized quickly by Smith and frequently encountered in the study of disease, was the problem of extraneous contamination. This was not considered to be an insurmountable problem by Smith:

> A minor difficulty, but one which may prove of more serious consequence to beginners, is the frequent encountering of bacteria other than those producing the disease in the organs of diseased swine. A perusal of the bacteriological observations in this report will show how much time has to be spent in isolating these bacteria and determining what relation they bear to the disease. Many of them can eventually be traced to the intestines where they commonly vegetate. Their presence in the internal organs may be accounted for by the extensive lesions in lungs and intestines which serve as entrances into the blood. This presence of strange bacteria has also been observed in other infectious diseases by other observers, and attention has been called to it in connection with hog cholera in the special report on that malady.[17]

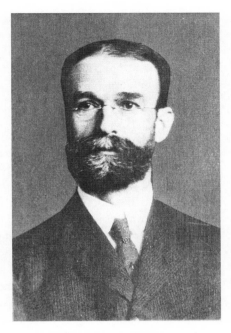

Theobald Smith (1859–1934), inspector within the Bureau of Animal Industry who first isolated the organism later termed *Salmonella*, named for Daniel Salmon, chief of the Bureau (courtesy National Library of Medicine).

As we see later in this book, similar problems were faced in attempting to identify the typhoid agent itself.

The authors of this book freely and extensively quote the early researchers in the field, believing this provides the most accurate means to understanding the thought processes of each individual as well as the understanding of their contemporaries. Hopefully the extensive use of contemporary material, much of it obtained directly from professional articles written by the scientists themselves, will appeal to the members of the audience interested in scientific history. We have attempted to limit, except where we feel it is necessary to develop the story, the use of scientific "jargon." One notable exception is Chapter 4, which deals with the etiological agent itself and describes in greater detail the pathogenic mechanisms associated with that agent. We believe this will be of interest to anyone wishing to understand the disease in molecular terms.

It is important to remember that the germ theory of disease is a relatively modern phenomenon. Prior to the 1870s, and particularly before the midpoint of that century, physicians generally had little idea of the relationship between proper sanitation and the outbreak of gastrointestinal diseases, as alluded to above. Certainly there were exceptions; the work of John Snow on cholera during the 1840s and 1850s is the classic example. Where these physicians demonstrated expertise in this area was in the reports of their observations, sometimes almost quaint in their descriptions, a belief with which we hope the reader will agree.

We would like to point out that neither of the authors is a professional historian. And while we would hope that members of the reading audience will include those interested in aspects of the history of medicine, the primary thesis of the book is that of medicine and not the background history of the period. There are no shortages of excellent histories available for the study of any of those subjects. For that same reason we have limited the use of statistics except where necessary in describing localized outbreaks, focusing on major participants—including victims as well as those who spent their professional lives studying the disease.

1

Earliest Historical Descriptions

Do not allow the army to use water that is unwholesome or marshy, as drinking bad water, just like poison, causes illness for the men.—Vegetius (*Epitoma Rei Militaris* [Summary of the Military] 1.22)

Perpetual springs within the walls are of utmost advantage ... but ... where nature has denied this convenience, wells must be sunk, however deep, till you come to water, which must be drawn up by ropes.—Vegetius (*Epitoma Rei Militaris* 4.10)[1]

In his late 19th century review of contemporary knowledge of typhoid fever, Heinrich Curschmann wrote what was clearly an understatement when referring to the historical appearance of the disease: "Typhoid fever, is, without doubt, <u>not</u> a disease which has developed or appeared for the first time within the last few centuries."[2] Part of the support for this statement is, by necessity, indirect. The ancients had no means to directly observe infectious agents or, for that matter, even to infer microscopic organisms as agents of disease. Confirmation of the existence of typhoid fever during that period has only recently been possible with the example of the Plague of Athens (430 BCE; see below). There is certainly no reason to think this was a unique outbreak for that period.

The most important specifically medical writings prior to the turn of the eras were those of the physician Hippocrates and his school. Hippocrates was born ca. 460 BCE in Kos, located in present-day Greece. During his lifetime, which lasted some 83 years, either he or his students composed what is known as the *Corpus Hippocraticum*, the Hippocratic Collection, consisting of some 60 medical treatises. Whether any of the illnesses described by Hippocrates actually represented typhoid fever can be debated. In his translation of Hippocrates' collected works,[3] W.H.S. Jones argues that the question of the existence of typhoid must remain an open question, but that the evidence would seem to suggest this was not among the illnesses Hippocrates described. Jones' argument was based largely on negative evidence, the absence of any description of anything specific to typhoid. As pointed out, Hippocrates dealt primarily with endemic disease, illnesses which formed the "background" of disease in those societies, rather than sudden outbreaks of epidemic disease. Hippocrates did refer to the presence of fevers, some of which were almost certainly malaria. However these fevers were described as not being "infectious," meaning contagious, as the term was then applied. Jones found this difficult to reconcile with what is known about typhoid. Yet Hippocrates generally applied that term in the context of the disease passing from person-to-person directly—colds certainly, but consumption (tuberculosis) as well. So here the question of whether there is any direct description of what is clearly typhoid must remain open.

What of the evidence that typhoid may indeed have been present during this time? Again the evidence is largely circumstantial. The symptoms of typhoid fever include development of a significant fever, dry cough, headache and abdominal pain. While certain symptoms of malaria may be held in common—headache and fever, the absence of a recurrent fever, often accompanied by periodic chills—would argue against that particular disease. In Books I and III of *Epidemics*, Hippocrates' description of the illnesses suffered by some of his patients certainly appears to be similar to typhoid.[4] In his descriptions, most patients became ill after drinking:

Silenus lived on the Broadway, near the house of Evalcidas. From fatigue, drinking and unseasonable exercises, he was seized with fever. He began with having pain in the loins; he had heaviness of the head, and there was stiffness of the neck. On the first day the alvine [intestinal] discharges were bilious, unmixed, frothy, high coloured and copious; urine black, having a black sediment[5]; he was thirsty, tongue dry; no sleep at night. On the second, acute fever, stools more copious, thinner, frothy; urine black, an uncomfortable night, slight delirium. On the third, all the symptoms exacerbated; an oblong distension, of a softish nature, from both sides of the hypochondrium [upper abdomen] to the navel; stools thin, and darkish; urine muddy, and darkish; no sleep at night; much talking, laughter, singing, he could not restrain himself. On the fourth, in the same state. On the fifth, stools bilious, unmixed, smooth, greasy; urine thin, and transparent; slight absence of delirium. On the sixth, slight perspiration about the head; extremities cold, and livid; much tossing about, no passage from the bowels, urine suppressed, acute fever.... On the eighth a cold sweat all over; red rashes with sweat, of a round figure, small, like *vari*, persistent, not subsid-

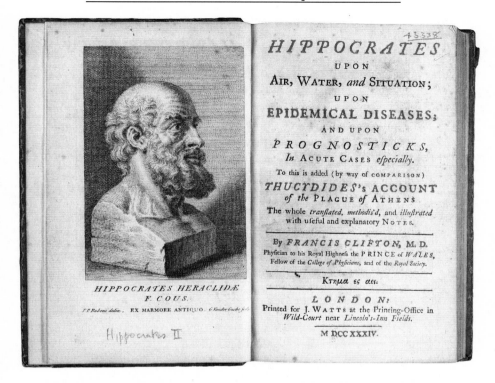

Bust of Hippocrates, 5th century BCE physician. Hippocrates was the first to describe what was likely typhoid fever (courtesy Wellcome Library, London).

ing; by means of a slight stimulus, a copious discharge from the bowels, of a thin and undigested character, with pain.... On the eleventh, he died. At the commencement, and throughout, the respiration was slow and large; there was a constant throbbing in the hypochondrium; his age was about twenty.[6]

Meton was seized with fever; there was a painful weight in the loins. Next day, after drinking water pretty copiously, had proper evacuations from the bowels. On the third, heaviness of the head, stools thin, bilious and reddish. On the fourth, all the symptoms exacerbated; had twice a scanty trickling of blood from the right nostril; passed an uncomfortable night; alvine discharges like those of the third day; urine darkish, had a darkish cloud floating in it, of a scattered form, which did not subside. On the fifth, a copious hemorrhage of pure blood from the left nostril; he sweated and had a crisis. After the fever restless, and had some delirium; urine thin, and darkish; had an affusion of warm water on the head; slept, and recovered his senses. In this case there was no relapse, but there were frequent hemorrhages after the crisis.[7]

In this case, the patient appears to have recovered. The absence of intermittent chills, or the return of symptoms, would argue against this being a case of malaria. Descriptions in Books I and III of *Epidemics* of similar illnesses would suggest that such cases even if not common were not exceptional either.

Similar cases were later observed by the Greek physician Aelius Galenus, more popularly known as Galen, who practiced his trade in the time of the Roman empire some six centuries later. Galen's descriptions of intermittent febrile illnesses certainly included that of malaria. Galen placed the fevers he studied into some five categories, based upon time intervals between recurrences: quotidian, tertian, quartan, semi-tertian (hemitritaeus) and irregular: respectively, daily, every second day, every third day, every second or third day (hemitritaeus), and periodically.[8] Victor Vaughan believed Galen's use of the term hemitritaeus (and Hippocrates as well) was descriptive of typhoid.[9]

Such descriptions of course fit those of any number of contemporary gastrointestinal diseases, particularly bacterial or amoebic dysentery. This does not even include possible viral infections or louse-transmitted illnesses such as typhus. The litany of illnesses likely would not include cholera, which if it did exist was more likely confined to the Indian subcontinent.

Disruption due to war and movement of armies certainly exacerbated the outbreak and spread of diarrheal illnesses. The Plague of Athens, almost certainly confirmed as an outbreak of typhoid fever, is discussed in a later chapter. But even earlier histories make note of gastrointestinal disease. Herodotus, the Greek historian who lived during the fifth century BCE, referred to such an outbreak in *The Histories*, in which he described the retreat of Xerxes and the Persian forces after their defeat by the Athenians in the Battle of Salamis [ca. 480 BCE]:

> All along their line of march, in whatever country they chanced to be, is soldiers seized and devoured whatever corn they could find belonging to the inhabitants; while, if no corn was to be found, they gathered the grass that grew in the fields, and stripped the trees, whether cultivated or wild, alike of their bark and of their leaves, and so fed themselves. They left nothing anywhere, so hard pressed were they by hunger. Plague too and dysentery attacked the troops while still upon their march, and greatly thinned their ranks. Many died; others fell sick and were left behind.... At Abydos [located in Egypt] the troops halted, and, obtaining more abundant provision than they had yet got upon their march, they fed without stint; from which cause, added to the change in their water, great numbers of those who had hitherto escaped perished.[10]

Several observations in the description by Herodotus are noteworthy. He had clearly made reference at least once—and possibly twice if we include the "change in water" at Abydos as contributing to the soldiers' miseries—

to a gastrointestinal infection. In the absence of a more complete description on the part of Herodotus, one can only speculate as to the nature of the illness; typhoid cannot be eliminated. In addition, given the flow of history, the defeat of the Persians would subsequently be numbered among the factors contributing to the Peloponnesian Wars between Athens and Sparta.

It has also been suggested that the illness suffered by Roman emperor Augustus Caesar in 23 BCE may have been either, or both, an abscess of the liver or typhoid fever. Although Augustus was expected to die, the story is that through the ministrations of his Greek physician Antonius Musa, who applied cold compresses or ice baths as a means of treatment, Augustus survived. As a means to honor Musa, a statue of the physician was erected and placed next to that of Aesculapius, god of medicine and healing.[11]

Epidemic disease was inherent in European civilization through the Middle Ages, roughly corresponding to the period from the collapse of the Roman Empire (~5th century CE) into the 15th century. The great increases in populations of larger cities, many of them confined by walls, and lack of proper sanitation procedures were primary factors in the outbreaks of disease during this millennial period. A possible contributing factor was that of diseases possibly introduced into Europe from explorers venturing into unexplored regions of the world; it has been suggested syphilis may have been such a disease. Wars were also commonplace during these years, with soldiers often the vectors of such diseases. According to the German historian Karl Sudhoff, eight diseases in particular were common: the Great Mortality (bubonic plague), phthisis (tuberculosis), epilepsy, scabies, erysipelas, anthrax, trachoma and leprosy. Sudhoff believed that what was diagnosed as either scabies or leprosy was probably syphilis.[12] The vague descriptions of these outbreaks, with the notable exception of the bubonic plague during the 14th century, make it a challenge to identify typhoid as the form of the malady. But several epidemics may very well have been this disease.

First, given the sanitary conditions that existed during these centuries and disruptions associated with the frequent wars, it is highly likely typhoid fever was among the diseases with which the citizenry was afflicted during this period. It is no surprise, however, that with the devastation wreaked by epidemics such as the plague, which may have wiped out as much as one-third of the population of Europe during the 14th century, illnesses such as typhoid simply became part of commonplace life in the cities. One possible outbreak of typhoid may have been the Neapolitan epidemic beginning in the winter of 1495 and lasting through the summer of 1496.

Descriptions indicate that during the Italian wars between 1494 and 1498, the French garrison left in Naples under the command of Charles VIII's viceroy, the Duke of Montpensier, and the Constable d'Aubigny may have nearly been wiped out by an outbreak of typhoid.[13]

There have been historians who question whether the epidemic was actually typhoid fever, or perhaps an outbreak of a virulent form of syphilis which might have been introduced into portions of Europe by this time. It has been suggested that syphilis may have been carried by Spanish troops who themselves had acquired the disease during Columbus's voyages to the Americas. The background to the Italian wars originated with the invasion in 1494 by French armies under the command of Charles VIII, who made claims to the throne of Naples. The invading forces included mercenaries from Spain, Germany and other regions of Europe. As has been common throughout history, the armies were accompanied by no shortage of "camp followers," and if sexually transmitted diseases were present there were plenty of opportunities for their dissemination. Ultimately the invading armies, including the French who had occupied Naples, were devastated by a disease of some kind and forced to retreat.[14]

The question is whether the disease could have been syphilis, or whether it was more likely typhoid fever. According to the British surgeon Professor Samuel Cooper, who provided an analysis of the outbreak, the disease had characteristics of a febrile illness likely transmitted through other than intimate contact:

> I think there must be infinite difficulty in coming to the conclusion, that the disease which broke out in the French army in Italy at the close of the fifteenth century, was the venereal disease, when you are informed that it spread among the soldiers so rapidly, and with such malignity, as to destroy in a short time a considerable part of that army. This is by no means the nature, or course, of the modern venereal disease; and, if it were, I suppose, it would thin our population more quickly than the present epidemic cholera. The venereal disease is sometimes attended with violent effects on the health, with terrible ulcerations, with afflicting pain and mischief in the bones and with other alarming and dangerous consequences; but it is not the nature of the disease to assume these aggravated forms in a sudden manner, or to destroy the patient in the rapid and unmerciful way displayed in the ravages of the disease which broke out in the French army at the siege of Naples. So far is this being the case, that it is one of the laws of the venereal disease for a certain interval, or, perhaps, I should say for an uncertain interval, should always transpire between the primary and secondary symptoms. Be it also remembered, that the disease which proved so fatal to the French army, could be transmitted from one person to another by breathing the infected air, by touching a sound part of the patient's skin, or

even by mere residence in the same chamber with him, without touching him at all. No complaint, having the characters here mentioned, would now be regarded as syphilis. In all probability, the disease in the French army was an epidemic febrile disorder, attended with ulcerations, buboes [swollen lymph nodes], abscesses, etc.; and at all events, it was a disease not resembling the modern "lues Venerea," which is slower and milder in its progress, not contagious, except by the application of matter containing the poison to the skin, or a mucous membrane; never sweeping off thousands at once in the rapid manner described by those who have detailed the particulars of the disease, which nearly annihilated the French army in Italy; and never extending itself through kingdoms and armies with the quick fatality, malignancy, and swiftness, noticed in the Neapolitan epidemic of 1495.[15]

Cooper's conclusion, which ignored in his argument the likelihood that sexually transmitted disease might indeed have been present in the mercenary armies and was probably spread throughout much of Europe once those armies dispersed, was that the Naples outbreak was a different disease than syphilis. The description would appear to rule out a respiratory illness such as influenza. The rapid spread and likelihood of poor sanitation would support the argument that this was typhoid. German historian Karl Sudhoff was equally emphatic in his belief the epidemic was not that of syphilis:

> It can be proved, from the travel notes of a German physician, that syphilis was not known in Barcelona [the alleged source of syphilis] in September, 1494; that throughout all Spain nobody mentions syphilis during the fall and winter of 1494, and at the beginning of the year 1495. Any extraordinary symptoms of a spreading epidemic were therefore not noticed in Spain until about the beginning of the year 1495!
>
> And what about the much heralded epidemic in Naples from March to May 1495? It is empty "historical" babble!
>
> Careful researches in the Neapolitan archives and in all the old chronicles leave no doubt as to this. Syphilis was not known there as a new disease before the beginning of the year 1496, and a general knowledge of syphilis was not established in the other parts of Central and Northern Italy before the spring of 1496; and this knowledge was partially, perhaps exclusively, spread by the little book of Scillacio, which left the press March 9, 1496, under the title: "*Novus morbus, qui nuper a Gallia defluxit* [The New Disease Which Had Recently Come from France]." For the frightful decimation of the garrison at Naples ... during the winter, spring and summer of 1495–1496, typhoid fever, and not syphilis, was demonstrably responsible.[16]

In 1635, some 150 years later, a febrile illness which appears to have been typhoid broke out among the soldiers in the French-Dutch army besieging Louvain during the midst of the Thirty Years War. The outbreak appeared to have been associated with ingestion of raw or unripe fruit and possibly contaminated meat as a result of the food shortages suffered by the attacking army.[17] At least 3,000 of the soldiers, possibly more, suffered from the outbreak, which became known as the French fever or French disease and which contributed to the subsequent retreat of the army (a similar designation was also used to denote syphilis).[18]

2

The Plague of Athens

The Peloponnesian War between the city-states of Athens and Sparta lasted over two decades, with what historians consider as three separate but interdependent phases between 431 and 404 BCE. The war became a defining feature in the development of ancient Greece. Details of the conflict are beyond the scope of this work, which will be limited to the early "highlights." Following the expulsion of the Persians in the first half of that century, Athens evolved into a commercial power backed by a strong navy. Sparta, allied with the Athenians in the wars with Persia, developed a powerful land army while becoming the chief rival to Athens. A series of revolts and battles among the (often surrogate) allies of each power subsequently resulted in war between the Spartans and the Athenians.

While outbreaks of disease certainly had taken place previously, the earliest "validated" epidemic is currently believed to have been that described by the Greek historian Thucydides in his account of the Plague of Athens (ca. 430–426 BCE) during the Peloponnesian War. The first year of the war, the region around Athens was occupied by the Spartan army, though Athens, under the command of Pericles and his sons, still maintained access to the water. Nevertheless, the invasion by the Spartans resulted in a significant proportion of the local citizenry entering the walled city and swelling the population. Estimates range from 250,000 persons to as many as 400,000, a number that undoubtedly overwhelmed whatever sewage system existed. According to Thucydides:

> In the first days of summer the Lacedaemonians [Spartans] and their allies, with two-thirds of their forces as before, invaded Attica, under the command of Archidamus, son of Zeuxidamus, king of Lacedaemon, and sat down and laid waste to the country. Not many days after their arrival in Attica the plague the plague first began to show itself among the Athenians. It was said that it had broken out in many places previously in the neighborhood of Lemnos [island off the coast of Greece] and elsewhere;

19

but a pestilence of such extent and mortality was nowhere remembered. Neither were the physicians at first of any service, ignorant as they were of the proper way to treat it, but they died themselves the most thickly, as they visited the sick most often; nor did any human art succeed any better.... It first began, it is said, in the parts of Ethiopia above Egypt, and thence descended into Egypt and Libya, and into most of the King's country. Suddenly falling upon Athens, it first attacked the population in Paraeus—which was the occasion of their saying that the Peloponnesians had poisoned the reservoirs, there being as yet no wells there—and afterwards appeared in the upper city, when the deaths became much more frequent. All speculation as to its origins and its causes, if causes can be found adequate to produce so great a disturbance, I leave to other writers, whether lay or professional; for myself, I will simply set down its nature, and explain the symptoms by which perhaps it may be recognized by the student, if it should ever break out again. This I can the better do, as I had the disease myself, and watched its operation in the case of others.

That year then is admitted to have been otherwise unprecedentedly free from illness, and such few cases as occurred all determined in this. As a rule, however, there was no ostensible cause; but people in good health were all of a sudden attacked by violent heats in the head, and redness and inflammation in the eyes, the inward parts, such as the throat or tongue, became bloody and emitting an unnatural and fetid breath. These symptoms were followed by sneezing and hoarseness, after which the pain soon reached the chest, and produced a hard cough. When it fixed in the stomach it upset it; and discharges of bile of every kind named by physicians ensued, accompanied by very great distress. In most cases also an ineffective retching followed, producing violent spasms, which in some cases ceased soon after, in others much later. Externally the body was not very hot to the touch, nor pale in its appearance, but reddish, livid, and breaking out into small pustules and ulcers. But internally it burned so that the patient could not bear to have on him clothing or linen even of the very lightest description; or indeed to be otherwise than stark naked. What they would have liked best would have been to throw themselves into cold water; as indeed was done by some of the neglected sick; who plunged into the rain-tanks in their agonies of unquenchable thirst; though it made no difference whether they drank little or much. Besides this, the miserable feeling of not being able to rest or sleep never ceased to torment them. The body meanwhile did not waste away so long as the distemper was at its height, but held out to a marvel against its ravages; so that when they succumbed, as in most cases, on the seventh or eighth day to the internal inflammation, they had still some strength in them. But if they passed this stage, and the disease descended further into the bowels, inducing a violent ulceration there accompanied by severe diarrhea, this brought on a weakness which was generally fatal. For the disorder first settled in the head, ran its course from thence through the whole of the body, and, even where it did not prove mortal, it still left its mark on the extremities.

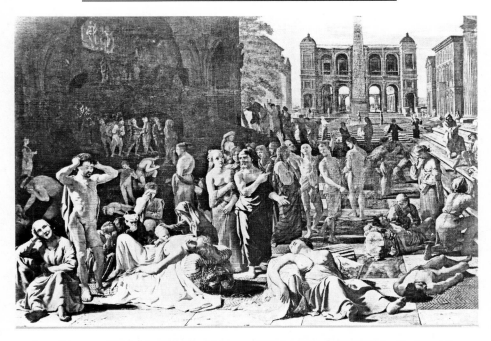

The Athenian Plague, by Nicolas Poussin. The painting clearly shows the suffering associated with the outbreak (courtesy Wellcome Library, London).

By the time the two to three waves of the epidemic had run their course between 430 and 426 BCE, approximately one-third of the population of Athens had perished, estimates ranging from 75,000 to 100,000 persons, including one-fourth of the Athenian army and its leader, Pericles.[1] Many of the victims were hurriedly buried in mass graves. There is no record of a corresponding outbreak among the Spartan army besieging Athens during these years, though the disease may also have been present elsewhere in the countryside (see above): "It first began, it is said, in the parts of Ethiopia above Egypt, and thence descended into Egypt and Libya and into most of the King's country."[2]

Historians have often speculated that the etiological agent of the epidemic could be any of a wide variety of diseases, ranging from influenza to smallpox, measles, typhus, typhoid and bubonic plague, even Ebola. Portions of Thucydides' description could be applied to any one of these or, just as possible, to none of them. For example, as part of a more recent series of analyses of disease outbreaks described in earlier histories, Burke Cunha compared Thucydides' description of the outbreak with symptoms associated with the most likely etiological agents: typhoid fever, typhus, smallpox and measles.[3] Characteristics described by Cunha included the acute onset of fever, the presence of pustules or ulcers Cunha referred to as a rash (here the translation is ambiguous and could as easily refer to blisters), sore throat accompanied by a dry cough, sleeplessness and subsequent death, symptoms which could be applied to any number of illnesses. Cunha also pointed out what appeared to be absent, or at least not part of Thucydides' description: convulsions, diarrhea—more about that below— and difficulty with vision.[4] In his summary, Cunha largely ruled out typhoid fever in favor of a diagnosis of measles or, less likely, smallpox. The absence of any spots or rash typical of smallpox would rule out that diagnosis.

Why did Cunha support the measles diagnosis rather than that of typhoid fever? The time of death following the onset of symptoms appeared less typical of typhoid: a week, as described by Thucydides, rather than the more common two to three weeks. The seeming absence of diarrhea was also a key point in Cunha's diagnosis. Yet Thucydides clearly included this symptom in his description of the plague: "the disease descended further into the bowels, inducing a violent ulceration there accompanied by severe diarrhea."[5] Cunha also pointed out that immunity to typhoid among survivors is uncommon, a characteristic applied to the outbreak by Thucydides as well. Yet clearly there was some immunity, albeit perhaps temporary: "Yet it was with those who had recovered from the disease that the sick and the dying found most compassion. These knew what it was from experience, and had no fear for themselves; for the same man was never attacked twice, never at least fatally."[6] Thucydides himself may have been a survivor.

There currently exists an effective vaccine against the disease, which of course was not in existence at the time of the plague. But what is the likelihood that surviving the illness would confer at least temporary immunity for the survivors? Studies have shown that natural immunity—that is, immunity which follows an acute infection rather than that from the vaccine—may persist as long as a year, declining significantly by that time. Effective gut immunity persists for at least that length of time.[7] This assumes the survivor does not receive a "booster" in the form of reexposure, an unlikely premise given the extent of the outbreak in Athens. One may conclude that the presence of immunity would not in itself rule out a diagnosis of typhoid fever. Nor can one rule out the possibilities that malnutrition, undoubtedly present in a city under siege, or a strain of bacillus more virulent than that found in modern times may have contributed to the outcome of infection. Cunha's primary arguments, including the high mortality rate, in favor of measles as the culprit could as easily fit any number of other illnesses. As Durack and his colleagues have pointed out in a blind analysis of Pericles as a patient, mortality among measles patients rarely has reached that level.[8] If one inserts the caveat that the citizenry in Athens represented a virgin population, it is conceivable that measles mortality could approach 25 percent. Durack's conclusion as to the etiological agent of the plague, based upon the description of symptoms provided by Thucydides, which included a rash of some sort, blindness, peripheral gangrene and the gastrointestinal and respiratory difficulties, was that the disease was typhus. The diagnosis is certainly within the realm of possibility given the overcrowding and unsanitary conditions; all that would be needed would be lice as vectors.[9]

However, the answer to the question of the etiological agent of the Athens plague has seemingly been answered using modern technology. The 1994 and 1995 excavations in Greece at the ancient cemetery of Kerameikos, a portion of which lay within the walls of ancient Athens, uncovered a mass burial site containing the skeletal remains of some 150 persons in five or more layers that could be dated to the time of the Athens plague. Authorities ruled out the possibility that these had been victims of the war itself, by the haphazard nature of the burial procedure: most likely these had been among the economically poor of the city thrown into a makeshift grave in an attempt to protect the remainder of the population from the pestilence.[10]

The ability to isolate and identify sequences of microbial DNA from ancient skeletons has produced a new area of medical forensics: paleomicrobiology. The principle is simple in its theory. DNA fragments are isolated from the source and amplified using the technique of PCR, the Polymerase Chain Reaction. Fractions which have been sequenced are then compared with modern counterparts available through an electronic database. The source material must be free from modern contamination, which could obviously skew the interpretation; hence care must be exercised when determining the location of the desired microbial material.[11]

Some of the skeletons had retained intact teeth, which allowed for the analysis of microbial genetic material which might have entered the dental pulp. Previous studies had shown that systemic infection by bacteria often resulted in microbes establishing an infection in regions of the dental pulp; the sites were considered ideal for such analysis, as they were generally protective against external contamination both during the life of the individual and following burial or later exhumation. Intact teeth were collected from three burial victims, with microbial DNA being extracted and shared among several independent laboratories for analysis.

Study of the microbial DNA resulted in the identification of *Salmonella enterica* serovar Typhi, the etiological agent of typhoid fever; no other potential forms of pathogenic bacteria were observed in the samples, providing strong support for the theory that the plague was an epidemic of typhoid fever.[12] This strain was a close relative of modern forms of the typhoid bacillus, with sufficiently slight differences to allow one to conclude this was an ancient strain. The obvious interpretation was that the Plague of Athens was the result of a typhoid outbreak in the city. Ironically, perhaps, this was exactly the approach suggested by Durack and his colleagues, which might theoretically solve the question. "There is the paleo-archeologic approach, in which archeological material is examined using modern techniques to establish a clinical diagnosis. The possibility of applying such an approach to the question of the cause of the Plague of Athens emerged last year [ca. 1999] as a result of the discovery in Athens by the German School of Archaeology of 160 skeletons dating to 430 BC. If scientific analysis of these bones using molecular techniques such as the polymerase chain reaction is successful, we just might find the answer to a question that has perplexed medical historians for more than 2 millennia."[13] And so we have.

3

The Strange Death of Alexander the Great

Given the overwhelming evidence that the Plague of Athens was probably an epidemic of typhoid, it is equally likely that the death of Pericles resulted from the same disease. One can provide a strong argument that another great military commander during that time, Alexander the Great, likewise succumbed to the same disease.

Alexander III of Macedon, better known to history as Alexander the Great, was born in Pella (present-day Greece) in 356 BCE, the son of Philip II, king of Macedon, and his wife (one of perhaps as many as eight) Olympias. Alexander had at least two siblings, a half brother, Philip III Arrhidaeus, son of Philip and Philinna of Larissa, and a younger sister coincidentally named Cleopatra. His mother and both siblings would later survive Alexander, albeit by only a few years in the case of his brother Arrhidaeus. Much of what is known about Alexander, including the circumstances of his death, comes from secondary sources written centuries later: the Greek historian Diodorus Siculus (ca. 90–30 BCE), the Greek historian Plutarch (ca. 45–120 CE), and Arrian of Nicomedia (ca. 92–175 CE). Writings by contemporaries of Alexander, particularly two of his officers, Ptolemy and Aristobulus, as well as the *Royal Ephemerides* (Royal Journals) written by Greek historians, possibly including the royal secretary Eumenes, during Alexander's lifetime may have been among the sources available to Plutarch and other historians. If so, they have long been lost to history.

Alexander has been remembered primarily for his generalship, the quality and success of which few would disagree about. But he was also a learned man, at least by the criteria of his times. As a young man he was tutored by the Greek philosopher and scientist Aristotle, whose works provided the basis for the natural and physical sciences and even medicine for over a millennium. For Philip (Alexander's father) the hiring of Aristotle logically followed the challenge of dealing with a son more likely to respond to reasoning than simply being ordered to accomplish a task. "A task for many bits and rudder-sweeps as well, he sent for the most famous and learned of philosophers, Aristotle, and paid him a noble and appropriate tuition-fee. The city of Stageira, that is, of which Aristotle was a native, and which he had himself destroyed, he peopled again, and restored to it those of his citizens who were in exile or in slavery."[1]

Philip was assassinated in 336 BCE by Pausanius, one of his bodyguards, the result of a perceived slight to the assassin. So at the age of twenty Alexander became king.[2] After settling a variety of scores, suppressing revolts on his northern frontier and eliminating potential rivals, Alexander embarked on a series of military conquests which would encompass most of the remaining thirteen years of his life.

Alexander's campaign into Asia began with crossing the Hellespont (now known as the Dardanelles) into the region of present-day Turkey in 334 BCE with an army variously described as consisting of between 50,000 and 55,000 soldiers and a navy approaching 40,000 men, primarily drawn from the city-state of Macedon. The dominant power in the east was that of the Achaemenid Empire, which had by then had existed for some two centuries. The ruler of the empire, Darius III, led an army larger than Alexander's. Nevertheless, this army was repeatedly defeated by the Greek forces. Darius himself was able to escape capture. Moving south through the Levant (eastern Mediterranean region), Alexander captured Tyre and Gaza, putting most of the males to death, and Jerusalem, which he spared. In 332 BCE Alexander occupied Egypt, where he was greeted as a liberator and proclaimed the son of a god.

The following year Alexander resumed his eastward pursuit of Darius, capturing first the city of Babylon—in present-day Iraq—followed by the Persian capital of Persepolis. Darius himself was subsequently betrayed and murdered by Bessus, one of the Persian satraps (governor) and cousin to the king, in 330 BCE.

As has been the situation in armies throughout history, among the challenges when on the march was the need for finding sources of palatable water, not only for the soldiers; during those thousands of years in which horses carried out much of the heavy work, water was required for the animals as well. This would have been true for Alexander's armies. Plutarch has included an anecdote relating not only the difficulty in obtaining fresh water, if one "reads between the lines," but also a description of the relationship between the commander and his men. While still in pursuit of Darius, one "which was long and arduous (for in eleven days he rode thirty-three hundred furlongs [nearly 400 miles]), most of his horsemen gave out, and chiefly for lack of water. At this point some Macedonians met him who were carrying water from the river in skins upon their mules. And when they beheld Alexander, it now being midday, in a wretched plight from thirst, they quickly filled a helmet and brought it to him. To his enquiry for whom they were carrying the water, they replied: 'For our own sons, even if we lose these.' On hearing this he took the helmet into his own hands, but when he looked around and saw the horsemen about him all stretching out their heads and gazing at the water, he handed it back without drinking any, but with praises for the men who had brought it; 'For,' said he, 'if I should drink of it alone, these horsemen of mine will be out of heart.'"[3] With water in short supply the army, which during these invasions comprised thousands of men marching through deserts, would likely drink from any rivers or streams they encountered regardless of possible contamination. Diarrheal diseases would merely represent one more form of occupational hazard.

In 329 BCE Alexander secured the northernmost portion of his empire with the defeat of a Scythian army in the Battle of Jaxartes, located near the modern city of Tashkent in the former Soviet republic of Uzbekistan. The battle is noteworthy for several reasons. Among those interested in Alexander's military conquests the battle represented the first known defeat of the nomad army. His benign treatment of the captured enemy removed any threat from that source to his further movements. An account of one portion of the battle provides further evidence for the ailment common to the soldiers: "[Alexander] put the Scythians to rout, and pursued them for a hundred furlongs, although he was suffering all the while from a diarrhea."[4]

By the winter and spring of 327 and 326 BCE Alexander's campaign brought him into the subcontinent of India. Following the defeat or subjugation of several opposing armies, Alexander reached the easternmost portion of his conquests: northern India near the Hyphasis River. By now his army had spent more than half a decade away from their homes and they threatened to revolt if Alexander decided to campaign any further. Unable to persuade his officers or men to continue, Alexander turned back. Two years later he again was back in Babylon.

Illness and Death

There are few certainties associated with the unexpected death of Alexander in the spring (June) of 323 BCE. That he been drinking heavily for some months is reasonably well documented, as it is corroborated by all accounts of his final year. The triggering event is open to speculation; it may have been grief associated with the sudden death of his friend (and lover), Hephaestion or the result of association with officers among his ranks who themselves indulged in drink. Regardless of the reason, his death occurred after a drinking binge at the quarters of Medius, a possible friend of Alexander's and commander of a trireme (a naval vessel), while entertaining Nearchus, who for a time was one of Alexander's satraps and later an admiral in his fleet. Since both Medius and Nearchus were associated with Alexander's naval fleet, it is entirely possible this was the basis for their association, if not friendship. "He [Alexander] laid aside his grief and betook himself once more to sacrifices and drinking bouts. He gave a splendid entertainment to Nearchus, and then, although he had taken his customary bath before going to bed, at the request of Medius he went to hold high revel with him; and here, after drinking all the next day, he began to have a fever."[5] It has been suggested by at least one contemporary of Alexander, Ephippus of Olynthus, that Alexander was "drinking the company's health in a twelve-pint cup."[6]

With the important caveat that each of the three most important descriptions of Alexander's final illness and death—that from Diodorus, Plutarch and, finally, the writings of Arrian the Nicomedian—may have drawn upon similar sources, it is useful to compare their respective works on the subject. Diodorus Siculus wrote as follows:

> They bade him sacrifice to the gods on a grand scale and with all speed, but he was then called away by Medius, the Thessalian, one of his friends, to take part in a comus [revelry]. There he drank much unmixed wine in commemoration of the death of Heracles, and finally, filling a huge beaker, downed it at a gulp. Instantly he shrieked aloud as if smitten by a violent blow and was conducted by his friends, who led him by the hand back to his apartments. His chamberlains put him to bed and attended him closely, but the pain increased and the physicians were summoned. No one was able to do anything helpful and Alexander continued in great discomfort and acute suffering. When he, at length, despaired of life, he took off his ring and handed it to Perdiccas. His friends asked: 'To whom do you leave the kingdom?' and he replied: 'To the strongest.' He added, and these were his last words, that all of his leading friends would stage a vast contest in honour of his funeral. This was how he died after a reign of twelve years and seven months."[7]

A portion of Plutarch's description has already been noted. Unlike Diodorus, Plutarch writes nothing about Alexander's having been subject to sudden pain upon drinking the cup of wine. In fact, Plutarch argued that any inclusions of a "sudden pain in the back as though smitten with a spear" were later inventions. Plutarch's further descriptions appear to have been based upon (no longer extant) original sources:

> In the court *Journals* there are recorded the following particulars regarding his sickness. On the eighteenth day of the month Daesius [June 2] he slept in the bathing-room because he had a fever. On the following day, after his bath, he removed into his bed-chamber, and spent the day at dice with Medius. Then, when it was late, he took a bath, performed his sacrifices to the gods, ate a little, and had a fever through the night. On the twentieth [June 4], after bathing again, he performed his customary sacrifice; and lying in the bathing room he devoted himself to Nearchus, listening to his story of his voyage and of the great sea. The twenty-first he spent in the same way and was still more inflamed, and during the night he was in a grievous plight, and all the following day his fever was very high. So he had his bed removed and lay by the side of the great bath, where he conversed with his officers about the vacant posts in the army, and how they might be filled with experienced men. On the twenty-fourth his fever was violent and he had to be carried forth to perform his sacrifices; moreover, he ordered his principal officers to tarry in the court of the palace, and the commanders of divisions and companies to spend the night outside. He was carried to the palace on the other side of the river on the twenty-fifth, and got a little sleep, but his fever did not abate. And when his commanders came to his bedside, he was speechless, as he was also on the twenty-sixth.; therefore the Macedonians made up their minds that he was dead, and came with loud shouts to the doors of the palace, and threatened his companions until all opposition was broken down; and when the doors had been thrown open to them, without cloak or armor, one by one, thay all filed slowly past his couch. During this day, too, Python and Seleucus were sent to the temple of Serapis to enquire whether they should bring Alexander thither; and the god gave answer that they should leave him where he was. And on the twenty-eighth [June 13], towards evening, he died.[8]

A similar detailed description of Alexander's final days was provided by Arrian, possibly from the same original source as that referenced by Plutarch.

> The Royal Diary gives the following account, to the effect that he reveled and drank at the dwelling of Medius; then rose up, took a bath, and slept; then again supped at the house of Medius and again drank far into the night. After retiring from the drinking party he took a bath; after which he took a little food and slept there, because he already felt feverish. He was carried out upon a couch to the sacrifices, in order that he might offer them according to his daily custom. After performing the sacred rites he lay down in the banqueting hall until dusk. In the meantime he gave instructions to the officers about the expedition and voyage, ordering those who were going on foot to be ready on the fourth day, and those who were going

to sail with him to be ready to sail on the fifth day. From this place he was carried upon the couch to the river, where he embarked on a boat and sailed across the river to the park. There he again took a bath and went to rest.

On the following day he took another bath and offered the customary sacrifices. He then entered a tester [i.e., canopied] bed, lay down, and chatted with Medius. He also ordered his officers to meet him at daybreak. Having done this he ate a little supper and was again conveyed into the tester bed. The fever now raged the whole night without intermission. The next day he took a bath; after which he offered sacrifice, and gave orders to Nearchus and the other officers that the voyage should begin on the third day. The next day he bathed again and offered the prescribed sacrifices. After performing the sacred rites, he did not yet cease to suffer from the fever. Notwithstanding this, he summoned the officers and gave them instructions to have all things ready for the starting of the fleet. In the evening he took a bath, after which he was very ill. The next day he was transferred to the house near the swimming-bath, where he offered the prescribed sacrifices. Though he was now very dangerous[ly] ill, he summoned the most responsible of his officers and gave them fresh instructions about the voyage. On the following day he was with difficulty carried out to the sacrifices, which he offered; and none the less gave other orders to the officers about the voyage. The next day, though he was now very ill, he offered the prescribed sacrifices. He now gave orders that the generals should remain in attendance in the hall, and that the colonels and captains should remain before the gates. But being now altogether in a dangerous state, he was conveyed from the park into the palace. When his officers entered the room, he knew them indeed, but could no longer utter a word, being speechless, During the ensuing night and day and the next night and day he was in a very high fever.

Such is the account given in the Royal Diary. In addition to this, it states that the soldiers were very desirous of seeing him; some, in order to see him once more while still alive; others, because there was a report that he was already dead, imagined that his death was being concealed by the confidential body-guards, as I for my part suppose. Most of them through grief and affection for their king forced their way in to see him. It is said that when his soldiers passed by him he was unable to speak; yet he greeted each of them with his right hand, raising his head with difficulty and making a sign with his eyes. The Royal Diary also says that Peithon, Attalus, Demophon, and Peucestas, as well as Cleomenes, Medidas, and Seleucus [officers and bodyguards], slept in the temple of Serapis [an Egyptian god], and asked the god whether it would be better and more desirable for Alexander to be carried into his temple, in order as a suppliant to be cured by him. A voice issued from the god saying that he was not to be carried into the temple, but that it would be better for him to remain where he was. This answer was reported by the Companions; and soon after Alexander died, as if forsooth this were now the better thing.[9]

Summarizing the accounts of Alexander's death—repeating the caveat that the two most detailed descriptions, those of Arrian and Plutarch, may have originated from an identical source (Royal Diaries)—the fatal illness appears to have originated following a feast in which wine was heavily imbibed. The illness lasted some eleven days, during which Alexander became progressively weaker and more ill. The illness was characterized by a high fever and subsequent loss of the ability to speak; whether this was the direct result of the illness or due to the progressive weakening of Alexander cannot be determined. One source, that from Diodorus Siculus, reported a sudden and severe pain—"he shrieked aloud as if smitten by a violent blow"—which Plutarch dismissed. The apparent absence of such in the description found in the Royal Diaries lends credence to Plutarch's dismissal.

The course of Alexander's final illness was provided in tabulated form by Burke Cunha. Descriptions of symptoms and comments largely originated from those in Plutarch and Arrian. The table that follows has been modified from Cunha and Philip Mackowiak.[10]

Dates (and Macedonian Calendar)	Symptoms	Comments
June 3 (Daisios 18)	Fever present	Bathed; slept in bath-house
June 4 (Daisios 19)	Felt "better" during the day, but that night the fever returned.	Bathed; sacrificed; ate a "hearty dinner; played dice with Medius
June 5 (Daisios 20	Fever increased	Discussed with Nearchus the upcoming campaign in Arabia
June 6 (Daisios 21)	Weakening as fever continued	Sacrificed; officers told to prepare fleet
June 7 (Daisios 22)		Transferred to house near bath
June 8 (Daisios 23)	Increased difficulties with sacrifice	Additional orders given to officers
June 9 (Daisios 24)	Speech began to fail (aphonic)	Carried from bed for sacrifices; officers told to remain in attendance
June 10 (Daisios 25)	High fever	
June 11 (Diasios 26)	High fever	Returned to palace
June 12 (Daisios 27)	Weakened and struggled to even raise his head	Troops filed past as Alexander watched

Dates (inc. Macedonian Calendar)	Symptoms	Comments
June 13 (Daisios 28)	Alexander dies during the evening	Allegedly minimal deterioration of the body prior to embalming six days later

What alternate explanations in addition to typhoid fever might address the symptoms described above? Two possibilities immediately come to mind. Given the political climate of the time, poisoning cannot be ruled out. Indeed, there was no shortage of adversaries, ranging from Antipater, the politically ambitious regent appointed by Alexander at the beginning of the campaign, to even Aristotle, his former teacher, who would benefit from Alexander's death. If Diodorus was accurate in reporting the sudden onset of (undefined) pain, poisoned wine could provide an explanation. However, the extended course of Alexander's illness would argue against this possibility. If one prefers to remain in the category of infectious disease, malaria is an alternate possibility. It was almost certainly endemic in the swamps of the region, and it is likely that Alexander had suffered from this illness earlier in his campaign against Darius. But here again the course of Alexander's fatal illness does not readily fit the symptomology of malaria. Alternative suggestions have ranged from West Nile to brucellosis to Guillain-Barré syndrome; but none clearly fit the description of Alexander's last days.

Several sources more strongly support the explanation of typhoid fever. Cunha has noted the presence of a continuous high fever, likely delirium and the extended period of his illness; the continuous fever, rather than one characterized by spikes, argues against malaria as a diagnosis.[11] Oldach and his colleagues, in a blind analysis of the symptoms, supported a diagnosis of typhoid fever largely through ruling out alternative explanations.[12] Mackowiak provided a comprehensive litany of Alexander's health problems during his campaign and came to an identical conclusion: the most likely explanation of Alexander's final illness was typhoid fever, possibly complicated by ascending paralysis and a perforated bowel, all of which are common to that illness.[13]

Is there additional evidence, albeit indirect, which would support the contention that the disease to which Alexander succumbed was typhoid? There may be, though none of the sources describe any contemporary outbreak of an illness with similar characteristics as that which killed Alexander. Alexander's "friend" and likely lover, Hephaestion, had risen in rank from Alexander's bodyguards to general of the cavalry, diplomat and even one of Alexander's most important engineers. The description of Hephaestion's death was similar in some ways to that described for Alexander a year later: "During this time it chanced that Hephaestion had a fever; and since, young man and soldier that he was, he could not submit to a strict regimen [arguably typical of young men even in modern times], as soon as Glaucus, his physician, had gone off to the theatre, he sat down to breakfast, ate a boiled fowl, drank a huge cooler of wine, fell sick, and in a little while died."[14] Alexander never fully recovered from the loss of his friend and continued to honor him until his own death. Poor Glaucus, Hephaestion's physician, was forced to pay with his own life for the failure to save Alexander's friend. The actual characteristics of the fever and the time span during which Hephaestion was ill are not described by the writers, but, in the absence of any evidence he had suffered from anything other than a disease of intestinal origin, it is likely this too was typhoid fever.

4

The Etiological Agent and Pathology

Previous chapters have provided examples of the earliest documented examples of possible typhoid fever outbreaks. Before proceeding further in developing the modern historical record of the disease—its identification as a unique clinical entity and the isolation of the etiological agent, each largely the result of research during the nineteenth century—it is useful to describe the actual organism and the human diseases with which it is linked. Two primary clinical conditions are associated with the genus *Salmonella*: salmonellosis or gastroenteritis, often referred to as salmonella infection or poisoning, and typhoid (enteric) fever, the focus of this book. Several less common clinical conditions may also be associated with members of the genus.

The naming of *Salmonella* species can be particularly confusing since nearly all the literally thousands of varieties in humans are in reality serological variations (serovars) of one of two human species: *Salmonella enterica* and *Salmonella bongori*. Genus and species names as applied to salmonella often represent the form of the disease, as in *Salmonella typhi*, or its site of isolation, *Salmonella newport*, rather than the more formal species and serovar designation. Hence the correct name for the typhoid agent is *Salmonella enterica*, subspecies *enterica* serovar *typhi*. To further confuse the student of nomenclature, *enterica* is one of six *Salmonella enterica* subspecies; subspecies *enterica* is in turn further subdivided into numerous serological variants, of which *typhi* is one. For simplicity, in recent history the etiological agent has often been designated as simply *Salmonella typhi* or *Salmonella typhosa*; older names included *Bacterium typhi*, or even *Eberthella typhi*. A series of similar serovars, *paratyphi* A, B or C (i.e., *Salmonella enterica* subspecies *enterica* serovar *paratyphi* A), are considered as the

34

etiological agents of paratyphoid fever, an enteric fever with characteristics similar to that of the more serious typhoid. To reduce confusion in this chapter we will simply refer to the typhoid bacillus as *Salmonella enterica* serovar Typhi.

Classification and Structural Characteristics of Salmonella

Members of the genus *Salmonella* are rod-shaped, Gram-negative bacilli placed in the Family *Enterobacteriaceae* (enterics), a group which includes the genera *Escherichia* and *Shigella*, each of which include species which are potentially pathogenic; despite the differences in names, at the genetic level the three genera are similar enough that one may conclude their evolutionary history included a common ancestor. As is the situation with all Gram-negative bacteria, the outer layer of polysaccharide—referred to as the somatic, O-polysaccharide or O-antigen—is among the determining factors for the designation of subspecies or serovar. Other surface antigens of significance include proteins associated with the flagellum (known as H antigens) or capsule (K antigens).[1] Because of its significant genetic flexibility, *Salmonella* has the ability to create thousands of combinations of surface antigens, the basis for the diversity designated as serovars.

While the determination of O and H variants among serovars plays an important role in identification of pathogenic strains of *Salmonella* involved in outbreaks, the actual pathogenic potential is associated to a greater extent with the presence of a capsule as well as other gene products informally designated as virulence factors. The capsule, called the Vi (virulence) antigen in *Salmonella*, is a surface polysaccharide; the genes associated with its synthesis are located on a pathogenicity island—*Salmonella* Pathogenicity Island-7 (SPI-7).[2]

Strains of *Salmonella* associated only with gastroenteritis generally lack SPI-7, suggesting that at least for initial intestinal infections the capsule may not be critical. The importance of the Vi antigen in the pathology of typhoid fever is not entirely clear since in the past a small minority of clinical isolates of *Salmonella* appeared to have been Vi negative; however, this may have been more a reflection of the sensitivity of the test than the complete absence of the capsule.[3] Whether or not its presence is a defining feature of typhoid fever, there is no question the Vi antigen contributes to the pathogenic potential using several mechanisms, beginning as early as the macrophage response. Repeated molecular patterns of proteins or polysaccharides known as Pathogen-Associated Molecular Patterns (PAMPs)

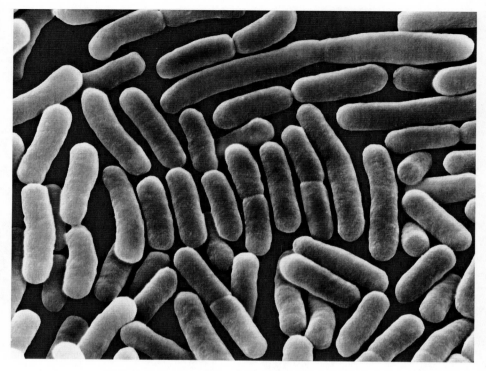

Salmonella typhi, **the etiological agent of typhoid fever (© Dennis Kunkel Microscopy, Inc.).**

on the surface of pathogenic bacteria are among the features recognized by immune cells and which contribute to the process of phagocytosis. The presence of the Vi antigen (capsule) is capable of masking those patterns on the cell, acting to inhibit phagocytosis.[4] If the organism is phagocytized the Vi antigen appears to interfere with both the activation of the phagocytic cell as well as interfering with internal killing mechanisms.[5] The interpretation from this is that the capsule may not be critical during the early stages of infection, as observed with strains not associated with typhoid fever, but may provide a survival mechanism for the more virulent strains (see below).

Infection and Penetration

While the initial stages of infection by *Salmonella* which result in either gastroenteritis or typhoid fever are similar, subsequent pathologies differ significantly. Other than pointing out that gastroenteritis is characterized by intestinal inflammation not generally found in the early stages of typhoid fever, descriptions of the infectious process and pathology associated with the organism will largely be confined to that of the latter.

Unlike many bacteria, strains of *Salmonella* associated with typhoid fever are confined to human hosts, including carriers with an inapparent or asymptomatic infection. The story of Typhoid Mary Mallon, described in a later chapter, is the classical example of such a carrier. Infection usually results from ingestion of contaminated food or water, a fecal-oral method of transmission.

The first barrier faced by the organism once it is ingested is that of stomach acid. *Salmonella* are highly sensitive to stomach acid and under normal conditions a significant "inoculum" is necessary for live organisms to pass into the small intestine. Anything which affects the level of stomach acid will obviously have an impact on the likelihood of such survival.

Once the organisms have passed into the small intestine or, subsequently, into the colon, they attach to the mucosal epithelium, entering what are referred to as the antigen-sampling microfold cells (M cells) for translocation across the epithelial layer. There is evidence the bacteria actually induce a transformation of epithelial cells into additional M cells, increasing the likelihood of penetration.[6] Additional physical changes take place as the bacteria contact the surface of the cells: a process referred to as "ruffling" occurs, in which alterations in the cell cytoskeleton take place causing the cell membrane to extrude and engulf the bacteria attached to the surface, analogous to phagocytosis.[7] The result is that bacteria are internalized in the intestinal cell. The process, sometimes called bacterial-mediated endocytosis (BME), is controlled by the genes located on a second type of *Salmonella* Pathogenicity Island: SPI-1. Among the polyglot of genes located on SPI-1 and involved in this stage of infection are those of a Type Three Secretion System (TTSS), needle-like structures on the surface of several types of pathogenic bacteria in addition to *Salmonella* which allow for the direct secretion of bacterial proteins into the target host cell.

Dissemination of *Salmonella* associated with typhoid fever begins with the uptake by phagocytic cells such as macrophage within the Peyer's patches, the bundles of lymphatic tissue associated with the intestinal mucosa. It is during this stage that the presence of the Vi capsular antigen may play a role in survival of the organism. Bacteria subsequently enter regional lymphatic tissue from which they may pass into the bloodstream for dissemination throughout the body.

Several possible clinical outcomes are possible during this period in an individual without additional underlying health problems (e.g., immune dysfunctions). First, even with the presence of the Vi antigen on their surface, disseminated bacteria may be eliminated by the host's immune system. Second, disseminated bacteria may be taken up by splenic or liver macrophage (Kuppfer cells) or cells within the bone marrow and mesenteric lymph nodes in which they may survive and multiply, with subsequent release back into the bloodstream in a secondary bacteremia. Intracellular survival of pathogenic strains of *Salmonella* appears to utilize a functionally distinct TTSS located on a separate pathogenicity island: SPI-2, the gene products of which block mechanisms of host cell killing.[8]

During the second bacteremia, bacteria may invade additional organs such as the kidney or gall bladder as well as reinfect gut mucosal cells, including the Peyer's patches. Damage to the intestinal mucosa is potentially more extensive, perhaps due to the reinfection process itself or as a result of an inflammatory response by the host. During this period the high fever and rash typical of serious cases of typhoid fever become apparent and may continue over a prolonged period of time, four to eight weeks in many cases. Bacteria may also be shed through fecal material or urine.

Infection and survival within the gall bladder, even in cases of typhoid which were inapparent, or at least mild enough to be missed in the diagnosis, plays a significant role in establishment of the carrier state. Bacteria may be released into the feces directly or survive within gallstones. The patient may not even be aware of the infection; approximately 25 percent of asymptomatic carriers had no previous history of typhoid fever,[9] and in preantibiotic days it was not unusual for the individual to be the source of an outbreak. Once again Typhoid Mary Mallon is the standard example.

The mechanism by which *Salmonella* survive in the gall bladder is uncertain. Obviously any cells which are within a gallstone itself are inaccessible to the immune system. In addition, there is evidence that bacteria within the gall bladder may begin production of a bile-mediated biofilm.[10] Biofilm production is a common process characteristic of many bacteria, particularly those which are potentially pathogenic, and is especially important in medical procedures involving catheters. There is an element of irony in a potential role played by bile in the environmentally induced production of a biofilm by *Salmonella* following penetration into the gall bladder. Bile is a mixture of water and bile salts—conjugated bile acids—produced in the liver and stored in the gall bladder, from which its release is important in the emulsification of fats during digestion. Because of its detergent-like characteristic, bile also exhibits antibacterial properties, and in fact is a component of some forms of selective media used in the laboratory to inhibit Gram-positive bacteria.

As is the situation in which environmental factors play a role in many aspects of bacterial pathogenicity, the mechanisms by which *Salmonella* resist the antibacterial properties of bile are not well understood. In fact, there are two overlapping aspects to the relationship between survival in the gall bladder with its high concentration of bile and its significance with respect to the pathogenic properties of *Salmonella*, roughly categorized as (1) mechanisms for survival in a bile-enriched environment, and (2) the induction of virulence properties as a result of exposure to bile.[11]

What has been learned about the first has largely been through indirect mechanisms: the use of genetic mutants in which relevant genes have been inactivated; correlations are described in which loss of specific genetic functions resulted in increased susceptibility to bile salts. A number of these genes have functions related to efflux systems, multicomponent protein complexes which transport, or "pump," deleterious substances such as antibiotics as well as bile salts from the bacterial cytoplasm to the outside of the cell. Among the most well-studied of these genetic systems in Gram-negative cells such as *Salmonella* is the acridine resistance (*acr*)*AB* complex, the products of which consist of several transport proteins and the outer membrane channel TolC.[12] Loss of this system or components within the system increase sensitivity to bile. The observation that mutants lacking this efflux system still retain partial resistance suggests other factors, including alternate pumps, may play a role as well.

The presence of bile also serves to regulate or activate virulence factors in certain Gram-negative infections including those of *Salmonella*.[13] Several of these functions appear to play a role in survival within the macrophage following phagocytosis, including modifications to the surface O-polysaccharides and resistance to host cell peptides. The common mechanism for seemingly disparate functions appears to be through the activation by bile of the PhoP-PhoQ (PhoPQ) regulon, a system which regulates the expression of several operon systems in *Salmonella* related to infection and survival.[14] As is readily apparent, *Salmonella* spp., not only *S. enterica*, carry out both an extracellular existence and intracellular survival critical to its disease capabilities. The PhoPQ regulatory complex appears to play a critical role in these stages of the intracellular/extracellular lifestyles of these organisms.[15]

As described above, bile may play a role in the positive regulation— i.e., induction—of certain genetic systems within the cell. It also appears to play a role as a negative regulator, the inhibition of expression of certain genes. For example, as described earlier, components of the SPI-1 pathogenicity island complex include a TTSS needle-like product which plays a role in the pathological effects of *Salmonella* penetration. The presence of bile has a negative/inhibitory effect on the expression of these genes, leading to a reduced level of invasion. The seeming dichotomy may be explained by the environment in which the organism may be found following infection. In the intestine, an environment in which the level of bile may be relatively high, invasion is reduced. Once the organisms have penetrated to the surface of the mucosa, bile concentrations are reduced and invasive mechanisms become more important. Based on this premise, Prouty and Gunn have proposed a hypothesis for initial events in invasion by *Salmonella*:

> We have formulated the following hypothesis of the role of bile in *salmonella* pathogenesis. After emerging from the stomach and entering the small intestine, the organism encounters bile released into the duodenum. While in the lumen of the anterior small bowel, the relatively high bile concentration represses the invasion pathway. Upon transit to the distal ileum, the luminal bile concentration will be reduced and the organisms will begin to transit the mucous layer covering the epithelium. Once within or beyond the mucous layer, the apparent bile concentration will decrease, allowing for derepression of the invasion pathway. Therefore, bile concentration may produce a signal allowing the bacterium to know if it was lumenal or close to the epithelium, where invasion factors must be synthesized.[16]

In addition to the effector molecules described above, as many as forty such virulence factors have been described for *Salmonella enterica* serovar Typhimurium, carried by a broad range of hosts in addition to humans, including fowl and rodents. Included among the virulence factors identified in this variant and secreted through the TTSS into the infected host cell are bacterial proteins which produce rearrangement of the cell cytoskeleton (actin), contribute to an inflammatory response and disrupt a variety of infected host cell functions; many of these are in a class of small *Salmonella*-encoded proteins called Pag proteins (PhoP-PhoQ activated genes).[17] It is unclear whether these proteins are among the virulence factors produced by the serovar Typhi and play any role in typhoid fever.

A summary of known or suspected virulence factors is presented in the table below and is adapted from Kaur (2012).[18] Most are encoded on so-called pathogenicity islands. The best known have been described above and are associated with the independently encoded TTSS located on SPI-1 and SPI-2. The role, or indeed the presence, of some of the factors in the pathogenesis of typhoid fever is uncertain.

Primary *Salmonella enterica* serovar Typhi Virulence Factors

Virulence Factor	Gene Location	Function
Vi (Virulence) antigen; SPI may also encode Type IV Secretion System and pilus	SPI-7	Surface polysaccharide: protection from phagocytosis; intracellular survival
Type Three Secretion System (TTSS); Effector proteins include SipA, B (*Salmonella* invasion protein), SopE (*Salmonella* outer protein), SptP (Salivary protein)	SPI-1	Translocation of virulence factors into host; so-called invasion genes; rearrangement of actin and cytoskeleton structure: ruffling; possible induction of apoptosis of macrophage
TTSS; Effector proteins include SpiC, SseF,G (secretion system chaperones), SspH2	SPI-2	Protection from host killing; intracellular survival and pathogenesis; disruption of vesicle transport; rearrangement of cytoskeleton
Magnesium transport system	SPI-3	Regulation of transport and genetic functions

The mortality rate among untreated typhoid victims ranges from approximately 10 percent to 30 percent; obviously the overall health of the victim will have an impact on these numbers. Populations which are undernourished—the situation today, for example, in third world countries where typhoid fever continues—would have a significantly higher rate of mortality. The underlying cause of death from typhoid appears to most often be attributed to severe bleeding associated with intestinal perforation, most commonly during the secondary bacteremia stage. It is possible this may result from the immunological response to infection. The descriptive pathology is that of ileocecal lymphatic hyperplasia, aggregated or enlarged lymphatic follicles, associated with the Peyer's patches. The process generally takes place about the time obvious clinical symptoms of typhoid fever begin to appear—one to two weeks, sometimes longer, after the original infection. Hyperplasia of tissues results in the projection of the region, almost resembling polyps, into the intestinal lumen, where necrosis and ulceration of the tissue may take place. The resulting peritonitis may become life-threatening, or, as is more often the situation in uncomplicated disease, over a period of one to two weeks the ulcers begin to heal. The cellular basis for hyperplasia is unclear, but as stated above, it may result from an overresponsive immune system. Those studies which have been

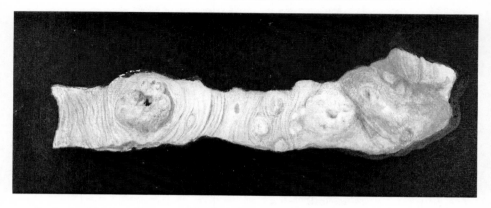

Intestinal lesions due to typhoid within Peyer's patches. The presence of such ulceration was critical in differentiating typhoid from other enteric fevers such as typhus (courtesy Wellcome Library, London).

carried out have focused primarily on risk factors rather than the actual molecular mechanisms controlling the response. Risk factors are largely nondescript. Ulceration is more likely to occur if the patient is male, has not been treated in a timely manner with antibiotics—obviously relevant only in the post-antibiotic era—and has exhibited leucopenia (low white blood cell count).[19]

What is understood is the nature of the cells which contribute to the hyperplasia of the lymphatic tissues. The majority of the immune cells which migrate into the tissue are mononuclear: lymphocytes as well as the more differentiated plasma cells, followed by macrophages, all likely the result of bacteria present during the second bacteremia.

Death of the immune cells, a process referred to as apoptosis or programmed cell death, and necrosis of the surrounding lymphoid tissue may be the result of the production and release of potentially cytotoxic chemicals by activated immune cells in response to the infection. In fact, it is highly likely that these immune cell cytokines are directly responsible for many of the pathological effects associated with typhoid fever, including the high fever, rash and cell death referred to above. These include Interleukins 1 and 6 (IL-1,6), Tumor Necrosis Factor-α (TNF-α) and members of the Interferon (INF) family.[20]

Even with the resolution of the illness, approximately 10 percent of (untreated) patients may become carriers, excreting bacteria for several months; a smaller proportion may become chronic carriers. By the beginning of the twentieth century physicians had become aware that in some carriers the responsible organ was the gall bladder, and cholecystectomy became a surgical option. In modern times the carrier state may usually be addressed with antibiotics.

Symptoms of Typhoid Fever

Infection is almost entirely the result of ingestion of contaminated food or water rather than person-to-person contact. The typical incubation period prior to the onset of symptoms lasts anywhere from one to two weeks, though instances have occurred in which the victim was asymptomatic for up to two months. During this period the primary bacteremia is taking place, and organisms may systematically spread throughout the patient. Symptoms which develop following the incubation period include:

- *Fever:* The temperature increases on a daily basis, reaching as high as 104°F by the second week. The fever may continue through much of the course of the illness, frequently accompanied by chills.
- *Headache*
- *Feeling of fatigue*
- *Rash* (usually on the abdomen and chest)
- *Cough*
- *Sore throat*
- *Constipation* (sometimes)
- *Abdominal pain* ("doughy" or distended).

During the second week after symptoms have appeared, if the disease is not treated the fever will likely continue. Abdominal pain often continues, and if intestinal perforation is taking place gastrointestinal bleeding will become apparent. If the illness continues into the third week the fever may continue and the patient may become delirious, lying almost motionless in what is sometimes referred to as the "typhoid state"; death may result. Jaundice is common if liver damage—death of hepatocytes—is taking place. If recovery is to occur the fever will begin to abate by the fourth week, though complete recovery may require months.

5

Scientific Progress in the 18th and 19th Centuries

It has been our common object to dispose a family of fevers, which have hitherto boasted of more than twenty names, under the simplest denomination and the most obvious specifical divisions. The genus then may be denominated *Typhus;* the species, gravior, mitior mitissimus, or febricula.—Edward Percival, Hardwicke Fever Hospital, Dublin.[1]

Percival's differentiation of fevers represented the early nineteenth century perception that all forms of fever were interrelated. The belief was understandable since, as pointed out by William Budd in his early review of the causes of that symptom, fever played a significant role in the practices of physicians in that era. Study of fever during the late 1790s and early 1800s had been initially influenced by the theoretical views of Herman Boerhaave (ca. early 1700s), a Dutch botanist and physician considered to be the "father of physiology" as a result of his work at the University of Leiden. Boerhaave was one of the first to attempt a classification of fevers. He described three forms of fever: "continued fever, ardent fevers and intermittent fevers.... He distinguished the autumnal intermittents from the vernal ones, a distinction necessary because of their different symptoms, duration and treatment. The autumnal intermittents resembled continued fevers in their onset, and Boerhaave recommended the prompt use of Peruvian bark for them."[2] Though his work represented only the views of his time, they provided a framework for observations carried out by physicians later in the eighteenth century.

Dr. William Cullen, a professor at the Edinburgh Medical School, one of the leading institutions in the medical field during the last years of the eighteenth century, modified the theoretical work of Boerhaave in attempting to incorporate the observations of contemporary physicians on the role of fever. Cullen was fooled by the lack of inflammation in some patients suffering from "fever," and while the presence of fever was clearly important in predicting the prognosis of an illness, Cullen believed that fevers were all interrelated. Cullen's views would significantly influence the thinking of those who followed him.

The establishment of "Fever Hospitals" attested to their importance. It was accepted by the physicians of the time that fever was a result of poor hygiene, but whether it truly represented a symptom of disease or was disease itself remained uncertain.[3] Classification of fevers during this period was largely influenced by two theorists: Thomas Bateman, physician of the London Fever Hospital, as well as, by consensus among his colleagues, the chief authority on diseases of the skin, and Edward Percival, quoted above. It was the belief of each that there existed a single form of febrile disease they termed *typhus*.[4] To Bateman and Percival, the classes of fever represented variations of the same disease.

But what was that disease as it is recognized in modern times—typhus or typhoid fever? The first clinical description of what is typhoid fever is generally attributed to British anatomist and physician Thomas Willis in his work titled *Of a Putrid Fever* (1659). Here is how Willis described the illness [spelling from the original]:

> In this Feaver, four times or seasons are to be observed, in which, as it were so many posts, or spaces, its course is performed: These are then, The Beginning, the Augmentation, the Height, and Declination. These are wont to be finished in some sooner, in others more slowly, or in a longer time. [Duration of the illness will vary among individuals.] The beginning ought to be computed, from the time the Blood begins to be made hot, and its Sulphur to conceive a burning, until the ardors, and burnings are diffused, thorow the whole mass of Blood [i.e., development of fever]. The Increase or Augmentation, is from the time, that the Blood being made hot, and inkindled thorow [hot throughout], burns forth for some time, and its mass is aggravated with the Recrements [saliva or mucus], or burnt particles, which increase the fermentation [i.e., increasing fever]. The state, or standing of the Disease is when (after the Blood has sufficiently burned forth and its burning now remits) the long vexed Blood, like a noble wrestler, when his adversary is a little yielding, recollecting all his strength, endeavors a bringing under, and a separation of that adust [darkened] matter [likely diarrhea], with which it is filled to a plentitude, and also, a Crisis or separation being once or oftener attempted, an expulsion of it forth of doors. The Declination succeeds after the Crisis or secretion, in which the Blood grows less hot, with a languishing fire, and either (the vital Spirit being as yet strong) overcomes what is left of that adust and extraneous matter and by degrees puts it forth, until it is restored to its formed vigour [the patient

lives]; or, whilst the same Spirit is too much depressed, the liquor of the Blood, is still stuffed with adust recrements, and therefore becomes troubled and depauperated, that it neither assimilates the nourishing Juice, nor is made fit for an accension in the heart, for the sustaining the lamp of Life [death].

Willis continued with a description of actual symptoms beyond that of the high fever: thirst, severe headache, abdominal pain, vomiting, diarrhea, and inflammation or rash.[5]

Thomas Willis (1621–1675)

Thomas Willis was born at Great Bedwyn in Wiltshire, the first of three sons born to Rachel and Thomas Willis. His father was the steward of the manor located there. His mother owned property in North Hinksey, Berkshire, and the family resettled there soon afterwards. By chance, the home was located a short distance from a private day school at Oxford, where the younger Thomas received his primary education. In 1637, he matriculated at the university in Christ Church, from which he received his bachelor's degree in 1639 and master's degree in 1642. During the English Civil War, which began that year, he joined the Royalist garrison at Oxford until its surrender four years later. In 1643 he published *De febribus*, an account of what was likely typhoid fever among the troops during the war.

In 1646 Willis received his medical degree, publishing his dissertation on the subject of "Fermentations, Fever and Urine." As already related, in 1659 he published the most detailed description for its time of what is likely typhoid fever. The following year, he was appointed Sedleian Professor of Natural Philosophy at Oxford, being granted the degree of doctor and shortly afterwards becoming a member of the Royal Society. After moving to London in 1667, he developed "the largest fashionable practice of his day," as well as becoming a Fellow of the Royal College of Physicians and receiving an appointment as physician to the king.[6]

During this period Willis carried out extensive research on the anatomy of the brain, including the classification of cerebral nerves, including the arterial circle at the base of the brain known as the "circle of Willis" [*Cerebrai Anatome/Anatomy of the Brain* (1664)]. Among the diseases and conditions he described were myasthenia gravis, puerperal fever and hysteria as a phenomenon which arose in the brain rather than the uterus. His publication *Pharmaceutica rationale* (1674) was considered one of the most important pharmaceutical works of the time. In it Willis described the significance of excess sugar in the urine of patients with diabetes mellitus, an important advance in the diagnosis of that disease.

One of the most bizarre events associated with Willis's career was the apparent "resurrection" of a woman believed to have died. In December 1650 a young woman named Anne Green was to be hung for the alleged murder of her son. It was likely the boy died as a result of premature birth. Nevertheless, Green was convicted of his murder. Following the hanging in Oxford, her body was brought to the home of Dr. William Petty, an anatomist at the university, for dissection and study. Willis and the other physicians noticed she was still breathing, and after several hours of treatment they managed to revive her. Green was granted a reprieve for the alleged murder and eventually fully recovered.[7]

Willis died in 1675 and was buried in Westminster Abbey.

Philosophical Views of Fever

As indicated in the preface for this book, in his edition of *Essay on Fevers*, published in 1739, John Huxham described a difference between "putrid typhus" (*febris putrida*)—typhus—and "slow nervous fever" (*febris nervosa lenta*—typhoid fever).[8] The distinction between the diseases was clear in his mind: "I cannot conclude this Essay on Fevers, without taking notice of the very great difference there is between the *putrid, malignant* and the *slow, nervous fever*; the want of which distinction, I am fully persuaded, hath often been productive of no small errors in practice, as they resemble one another in some respects, though very essentially different in others."[9]

There was precedence for Huxham's attempts to distinguish between the two forms of illness. Dr. Ebenezer Gilchrist of Dumfries, in his *Essay on Nervous Fever* published in 1734, described the symptoms of nervous fever as including "diarrhea, abdominal pain, melaena [blackish feces indicative of intestinal bleeding], epistaxis [nosebleeds], partial sweats which gave no relief, and in the advanced stages delirium, and other cerebral symptoms.... I take this fever to be very different in its nature and changes from other fevers."[10] Dr. Browne Langrish of London, in a work published in 1735, also distinguished between the two forms of fever, noting that the illnesses described as *Slow Nervous Fevers* were characterized by "a quick but variable pulse, vomiting, purging, and a duration from twenty to thirty days." In his discussion, Langrish also objected to two of the more common forms of treatment: bleeding and purging.[11]

While numerous physicians during the latter half of the eighteenth century observed a distinction between the enteric fevers (typhoid and typhus) based on the form the fever would take, it would be in the first decades of the new century that the diseases were clearly distinguished on the basis of their respective pathologies. During this period, France emerged as the focal point of medical research. The French Revolution, which began in 1789, had gutted the old political system, bringing with it both institutional changes and changes in the way physicians thought about diagnosis and treatment. Fueled by Enlightenment ideas of reasoning, experimentation and questioning of long-held assumptions, several of the physicians who worked, or were trained, in France were able to shed light on the identification and diagnosis of typhoid fever.

Following the revolution, French hospitals that had been owned by the church were nationalized. Originally, revolutionaries had actually intended to eliminate the hospitals altogether. As industrialization had brought people to the cities, hospitals had become horrifically overcrowded and mismanaged. It was not unusual to find multiple patients sharing the same beds and living in filth. Tenon believed "the general policy of the Hôtel Dieu—policy caused by the lack of space—is to put as many beds as possible into one room and to put four, five, or six people into one bed. We have seen the dead mixed with the living there.... Often we have seen contagious and noncontagious diseases in the same wards, women with syphilis and some with fever. The operation ward where they trephine, cut the stone, and amputate members contains those who are being operated upon, those who will be operated upon, and those who already have been operated upon.... The St. Joseph ward is designated for pregnant women. Legitimate spouses and whores, healthy and sick women are all together. Three or four are in the same bed, exposed to insomnia, contagion, and the danger of hurting their children. The delivered women are also four or more in the same bed at different periods after delivery. It is nauseating to think how they infect each other. Most of them die or leave diseased."[12]

Instead of abolishing such hospitals, officials decided to reform the system. Some basic measures they introduced involved the enlargement of existing hospitals, constructing new hospitals, and separating the sick from prisoners or other poor persons. In Paris, hospitals became known not only for their centralization and efficiency, but also for instituting internship programs and placing physicians on the same level as surgeons.[13] These hospitals and the people that staffed them emphasized clinical experience—examining both the living and the dead—whereas their predecessors had relied largely on tradition and book learning.

Among the most important figures behind this change in philosophy was Pierre Cabanis. Cabanis graduated with a medical degree in Paris in 1783. One of his patients was Honoré Gabriel Mirabeau, among the early leaders of the French Revolution in 1789. Plagued by ill health, Mirabeau died in 1791, and Cabanis himself barely survived the excesses of the revolution. He spent most of the 1790s in philosophical pursuits, even helping draft the proclamation for Napolean Bonaparte's coup in 1799.[14] In the years which followed, Cabanis returned to his work in medicine while maintaining a larger philosophical approach to the subject. He published several books dealing with topics such as medical education and hospital reform. In Cabanis' view, all good medicine boiled down to observation: "The true instruction of young doctors is not received from books, but at the sickbed."[15] In many ways, this was a significant departure from reliance on traditional modes of thinking prerevolution, though Cabanis continued to believe in the Hippocratic view of four temperaments—sanguine, choleric, melancholic and phlegmatic—in controlling human health and behavior. He opposed the notion that new treatments might be necessary in dealing with disease, maintaining "we don't need new remedies; we need only a good method of using those we have."[16] Cabanis' significance, however, was due to his emphasis on pragmatic action, a philosophy which encouraged others to search for evidence and to avoid being trapped by unsupported theory.

The school of thought embraced by Cabanis, that of empirical evidence, would come to dominate the medical community in Paris. It could arguably be summed up by a phrase Jean-Nicolas Corvisart, perhaps the most important of the early French cardiologists and personal physician to Bonaparte, had engraved on his lecture room wall: "Never do something important following pure hypothesis or simple opinion."[17]

Johann Valentin von Hildenbrand and "Contagious Fever"

One of the many reasons for confusion over how to define typhoid was the existing terminology. The term typhus continued to be used generically in designating a variety of fevers. In 1810 Johann Valentin von Hildenbrand, professor of practical medicine at the University of Vienna, published a treatise in which he attempted to clarify the definition of typhus. In doing so, Hildenbrand was unknowingly antedating the subsequent work of the French and English (British and American) schools of thought on the subject:

[Hildenbrand argued that the designation of typhus was] improperly employed to designate a *genus* of disease, and that it ought to be used as the name of a particular *species....* The true typhus has often been mistaken for another fever [typhoid, a name not yet coined in 1810?], just as certain other fevers have been mistaken for typhus. In order to avoid all further dispute about the name of a disease of which the primitive meaning has been lost by an abuse of language, I declare that I treat in this work of the true *contagious typhus* [likely "true" typhus as later defined by William Gerhard] alone, which develops in the human body its special poison by means of which it afterwards spreads, which is everywhere and always perfectly like itself, and of the same essential nature, because it proceeds from a poison *sui generis* [unique] and always the same, which disease in fine ought alone to bear the name of typhus because it possesses the special characters expressed by that word. Contagious typhus is an essential fever the course of which displays a constant uniformity. It is a fever of a *special species*—as small-pox, for example. It is contagious because by means of a special substance which develops during the disease it is transmitted and communicated to those who are predisposed to it. By reason of an eruption which is peculiar to it, it belongs to the family of the exanthematic fevers, among which the contagious fevers ordinarily find their place [italics in original].[18]

In his treatise, Hildenbrand (almost correctly) explained the mode of transmission of contagious typhus: "The mediate contagion, then, may be communicated in numerous ways; but most commonly by articles of clothing, such as linen stuffs, furs, dirty bed-clothes, and even by means of the straw or the skins, upon which the patient may be obliged to lie during his illness."[19] The role played by the body louse in transmission of (true) typhus would not be shown for generations. But it is clear Hildenbrand was able to distinguish typhus from other forms of "nervous" fevers, including typhoid (see also *n*8).

Distinguishing Enteric Fevers: Bretonneau and Louis

The school of thinking embraced by Cabanis, Corvisart and others led to an evolution in thinking about diseases such as typhoid. Two French physicians in particular, Pierre Bretonneau and Pierre-Charles-Alexandre Louis, were able to apply the presence of fever in combination with their studies of intestinal lesions in differentiating typhoid fever from other enteric fevers.

As a student, Pierre Bretonneau attended lectures presented by Corvisart, who was then a professor at the College of France. Corvisart's influence on Bretonneau's approach to the study of disease would play a significant role in the latter's study of typhoid. After obtaining his degree in 1814, Bretonneau served as a physician at the hospital in Tours. Much of his practice was found in the rural areas of the region, allowing him freedom to observe and study epidemics in those areas. The first of these outbreaks which he experienced occurred in 1802 while Bretonneau was the young mayor of Chenonceaux, a small town some miles east of Tours. Similar outbreaks took place in 1812 and in Tours again in 1819. Similarities in these epidemics led Bretonneau to suspect all had an identical cause.

As described by William Budd in his review of enteric fevers, rural epidemics demonstrated features which would not normally be available in a more urban setting. The patient or victim rarely develops the same illness more than once, while the spread of the disease from person to person speaks of its contagious nature.[20] Bretonneau was in an ideal situation for his analysis of the 1819 outbreak in Tours. He had already had experience in the study of earlier outbreaks while at Chenonceaux. As a medical officer at the hospital in Tours, he would have had access to the bodies of victims for postmortem studies as well as the ability to compare any observations with those found in individuals dead from other causes. In effect, these other individuals could serve as controls.

Bretonneau carried out over 300 autopsies on humans and nonhuman animals during these years, including 120 on persons who died of "fever."[21] In 1820 he first reported that the ulceration and inflammation associated with typhoid was located primarily in the Peyer's patches, the lymphatic glands of the ileum portion of the small intestine. His analysis included the differentiation of this disease from others which might also produce forms of ulceration in the intestine, such as dysentery or tuberculosis. Furthermore, the disease was always localized in this region of the intestine, its presence unrelated to the severity of the illness.

While Bretonneau recognized the contagious nature of the disease, he was convinced the agent was a poison of some sort which somehow spread from person to person and resulted in a form of inflammatory reaction. Because the ulcerations appeared to him as a tumor or pock, he named the condition dothienenenteritis, or "tumor or boil of the intestine." While Bretonneau first described these observations in 1819 and 1820, it was only after his student Armand Trousseau published the work in 1826 that it became widely known, and he received proper credit for the discovery. Bretonneau himself published a more thorough account shortly afterwards.[22]

It is unknown exactly why Bretonneau chose to defer the report of his observations. Budd has speculated the delay may have been in part the contrast between Bretonneau's analysis of a specific epidemic—that of

1819—and the wider experience of other physicians in Paris. While they fully accepted Bretonneau's observations in what initially involved a small number of postmortems, it was more difficult for them to believe the lesions could be used in defining "a specific febrile disease."[23]

Trousseau's decision to publish Bretonneau's work in 1826 may have been the result of fear on the student's part that competitors might argue priority in their observations. Trousseau wrote as follows in his 1826 report:

> Before now works on pathological anatomy and clinical medicine have described perfectly the various changes in the inner gastro-intestinal membrane. The works of Broussais, Petit, Serres, Rayer, Andral, Hutton, Leuret and Billiard, have accurately pointed out to us the different forms in which inflammation can appear in the digestive tract, but there is something lacking, it seems to me, since none of these authors have attached in a precise fashion a series of symptoms to certain changes; thus under the name of gastritis, enteritis, colitis, vollitis, erythematous, erysipelatous, aphthous and postulant inflammation, etc., we have confused each in turn and no one has determined but very imperfectly, the common symptoms, or the differential signs of each of these inflammations, moreover, it is possible that the internal tegument, as well as the external, is subject to different and specific inflammation.
>
> The long and useful work of Dr. Bretonneau has finally cleared up this question. Since 1813 he has collected a large number of cases in his civil practice, as in the hospital at Tours, at whose head his merits have placed him.
>
> He has been led to distinguish a disease, the seat of which appears to be exclusively in the glands of Peyer and Brunner [Peyer's patches], which one finds in the jejunum, ileum [primarily] and large intestine. He has given this affection the name of dothinenteritis. He has indicated the relationships, traced the symptoms and described with precision, the appearance of the disease, which changes on successive days. He has stressed so well, all of the essentials of the diagnosis, that few of his pupils, or of the great number of those who have had knowledge of his researches and ideas, cannot distinguish perfectly well in most cases, from all other forms, this form of enteritis which is so common.... I wish to give a sketch of his [Bretonneau's] labors in order to call the attention of physicians to a disease extremely frequent, but hardly studied until the present, *and also to ensure Dr. Bretonneau the possession of his discovery which they have already wished to take from him* [italics added].

Budd believed the "they" were likely either Pierre Louis or any of a number of other physicians carrying out work similar to that of Bretonneau.[24] In his report, Trousseau described the day-to-day changes which took place in the glands of Peyer and Brunner as the disease progressed. It was Trousseau's (and Bretonneau's as well) argument that "in indicating, during this short exposé, the anatomic lesions characteristic of [doth]inenteritis,

I would not wish to say that the gland of Peyer or of Brunner were exclusively affected, but I say and that is what the most careful observation has shown M. Bretonneau, that if in dothinenteritis, the stomach, the small intestine, and the large intestine, have been found sometimes inflamed, independent of the glands of Peyer and Brunner, this inflammation cannot be considered other than an accident which does not hinder this latter disease from taking its course and from presenting the symptoms which characterize it."

Pierre-Fidèle Bretonneau (1778–1862)

Pierre-Fidèle Bretonneau was born in Saint-Georges-sur-Cher, the son of a local surgeon and nephew of another. A medical career was almost foreordained in that, over nine generations, his family had included fifteen members of the medical profession. His medical studies began in 1795 in Paris, where he entered the École de Santé. His studies were financed by a Madame Dupin, whose lecturer he subsequently married. Ill health forced Bretonneau to discontinue his studies and return home. He made another attempt at completing his work in 1799 after returning to Paris but failed to pass his doctorate examination. Instead he received the title of "officier de santé," a level below that of doctor or surgeon.[25] Bretonneau then returned to Chenonceaux to practice. In 1803 he became mayor of the town, serving in the capacity until 1807, during which time he had the opportunity to observe the aforementioned epidemic.

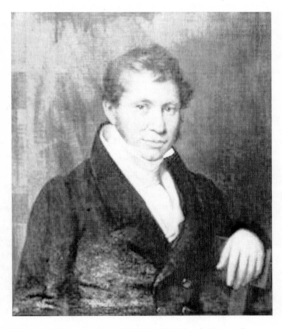

Pierre Bretonneau (1778–1862). A French physician, Bretonneau is credited with observing that specific symptoms of enteric fevers were due to typhoid fever, thereby identifying that disease. Bretonneau was also the first to identify diphtheria. His work and interpretations were forerunners of the Germ Theory of Disease (courtesy Wellcome Library, London).

Bretonneau spent fifteen years at Chenonceaux. In 1814, he finally passed his medical examination and obtained his degree. Afterwards he moved to Tours, where in 1819 he became chief physician, a position he held for 23 years. His studies of local epidemics entailed more than what was established as typhoid fever. In 1819 an outbreak of an illness characterized by severe sore throats and high mortality broke out. Bretonneau performed autopsies on 60 victims, noting a similar pathology, and proposed the name "diphtheritis" for the disease.[26]

He spent much of the decade of the 1820s studying what we now recognize as typhoid. Among his most important students during these years were Trousseau and Alfred Armand Velpeau, each to become prominent in his own right. Bretonneau's insistence that typhoid and diphtheria (to use the modern terminology) were specific diseases, likely associated with specific agents, was confirmed once the germ theory of disease was established a generation later. His work was at times hampered by the lack of technology. Not least among the challenges he faced in researching the causes of disease was the difficulty in obtaining a microscope. Bretonneau died at the age of 84, six years after a second marriage—this time to an 18-year-old woman.

Trousseau had reason for concern in his determination that Bretonneau should receive priority for his studies of enteritis. The other notable French physician simultaneously carrying out similar studies, Pierre Charles Alexandre Louis, had made comparable observations in the small intestines of persons dying from typhoid and published those observations in two volumes in 1829: *Recherches anatomiques, pathologiques et thérapeutiques sur la maladie connue sous les noms de gastro-entérite, fièvre putride, adynamique, ataxique, typhoide, etc.* [Anatomical, pathological and therapeutic research on the disease known under the names Gastro-enterite, Putrid, Adynamic, Ataxic or Typhoid Fever, etc.][27] The publication represented the culmination of nearly a decade of work on Louis's part in examining intestinal perforations.

In particular, Louis drew his conclusions following the postmortem examination of ten patients who had died following perforation of the ileum. The illness in nine of the ten cases began with a mild fever and diarrhea and subsequently progressed to include symptoms of rash, increasingly severe abdominal pain—no doubt the result of perforation—delirium and eventual death. Upon postmortem examination of the bowel, Louis observed the lesions within the Peyer's patches. While he described the illness as *Fièvre typhoide*—typhoid fever—coining the name in the process, Louis did not differentiate that malady from typhus, an illness which in fact was not present in Paris at the time.[28] Louis observed that most of the persons in Paris who succumbed to this fever were young and new to the city. He felt this supported the contention that the disease was contagious, despite the denial by other physicians in the city, and that this population was particularly vulnerable since they had not been previously exposed. His response to the denial was that since the disease had broken out in a large city, it was difficult to trace an actual source.[29]

In the second edition of his treatise (1841), Louis provided strong evidence for not only the source of typhoid, but also its contagious nature. One patient, termed Observation 54, became ill following the likely ingestion of putrid water contaminated with chopped-up hay. This "was followed by a well-developed and fatal case of typhoid fever in which the ulcerations of the Peyer's patches were found after death."[30] Dr. Esprit Gendron of Château-du-Loir had used the information obtained from repeated epidemics of typhoid in small villages to come to similar conclusions about the contagious nature of the disease: "While everyone accepts the contagiousness of smallpox, measles, scarlet fever, and even dysentery, typhoid epidemics are invariably ascribed to climactic changes or to the 'constitution—i.e., to infection (through the air) rather than contagion. But after observing a series of cases where families sleeping together in the same bed passed typhoid to one another, Gendron concluded that it spreads by contagion, 'poisoning by an unknown and impalpable principle known as a miasm.'"[31]

Utilizing observations from the 1834–1835 epidemic provided by Gendron, Louis used those examples to argue in favor of both "direct and indirect transfer" of typhoid between victims as well as "immunity [being] conferred by an attack of the disease:

1. Three journalists contracted the disease at a certain house; two communicated it to their families; the third did not do so, he was looked after by his wife who had had the disease several years before.

2. A domestic servant of Contereau transmitted typhoid fever to his sister, the niece of his master and mistress, and these visited her without danger. They had had the typhoid affection four years before.

3. At Petit-Gênes a young man infected all who looked after him except his father and mother; these had both previously had dothinentérie; the husband 20 years and the wife two years before the epidemic which this very son started.

4. In 1829 the same disease was imported into a fresh family at Petit-Gênes and did not go beyond it, in spite of the visits of the inhabitants of the hamlet, which had already been once attacked.

5. At eight years apart two epidemics attacked Coemont and the second spared all those whom the first had not spared.

[Louis concluded with] It seems to me henceforth impossible, after all that goes before, to deny the contagious character of the typhoid affection, even in Paris.[32]

It should be pointed out that at the time none of the French physicians could definitively differentiate between the two diseases despite the differences in their respective pathologies. In part, the difficulty lay in the inability to carry out extensive postmortem examinations of typhus victims since, as noted earlier, the disease was less common in France.

Pierre-Charles-Alexandre Louis (1787–1872)

During the early decades of the nineteenth century—a period in which young men from any country interested in a medical career gravitated to France, none were more inspiring or influential to these aspiring physicians than Pierre-Charles-Alexandre Louis.[33] Louis was born in Ay, Champaign, the son of a wine merchant. Though initially interested in a career in law, he decided instead to study medicine. After beginning his studies at Reims, he moved to Paris, where he received his medical degree in 1813. At the time, a common theme among many young French physicians was what became known as "therapeutic skepticism," or "nihilism," the view that nature should be allowed to cure disease rather than through the use of medications by doctors. Unsure of how to utilize his degree, Louis accepted an offer by a friend, the Comte de Saint-Priest, to travel to Russia where he could obtain experience in his profession. After traveling for three years he settled in Odessa (1816), where he developed a practice, even obtaining the honorary title of physician to the czar. Dissatisfied with the methods available in treating disease, particularly during a diphtheria epidemic which broke out there, Louis returned to Paris in 1820 and obtained a position as assistant to Dr. Auguste-François Chomel, professor of clinical medicine. He would spend the next six years working and living at La Charité Hospital.

It was while working in the hospital system in Paris that Louis honed his techniques. First was the importance of observation, or "exact observation" as some called it: actually questioning and listening to each patient. As he described it, *Ars medica tota in observationibus*—the art of medicine is all in observation."[34] Louis took methodical notes so that he could perform statistical analyses on his data. As pointed out by one of his biographers, the 1820s represented one of the heights of statistical analysis. Pierre Simon de Laplace had developed a system of statistical correlations and Louis adapted this method of analysis in his study of disease.[35] Louis' first major application of statistical analysis was in his study of tuberculosis. The French physician Rene Laennac had carried out an extensive study of that disease shortly after the beginning of the century. But the various manifestations of the illness had made analysis of morbidity and mortality rates a challenge. Louis, beginning with 123 patients of his own who suffered from tuberculosis, detailed the symptoms and lesions and, adapting Laplace's methods of analysis, came up with numerical/statistical conclusions for the study of the disease. His work, *Recherches anatomico-pathologiques sur la phthisie (Pathological Research on Tuberculosis)*, which was published in 1825, continues to be one of the most significant analyses on that subject.[36] His volumes on typhoid published in 1829 and 1841, as described above, represented a significant achievement towards understanding that disease. Louis's statistical analysis of the use of leeches for bloodletting in the treatment of diseases such as pneumonia, a technique championed by François Broussais (see n26) demonstrated the uselessness of that technique.

But it was Louis's training of students that produced the greatest impact in medical knowledge. In addition to Gerhard, Pennock and Shattuck, his protégés included Oliver Wendell Holmes of Boston, who helped demonstrated that puerperal fever in women was the result of unsanitary practices; and Henry Bowditch, a physician, prominent abolitionist and future president of the American Medical Association. Louis, who later in life married the sister of writer Victor Hugo, died at the age of 85.

Concluding the Story

The confusion was resolved independently by British and American physicians. As became apparent later, both typhus and typhoid fever were present in Britain, the incidence of the former being greater than that found in France, where typhus was rare. Beginning in 1825 and carrying over into the following year, an epidemic of fever broke out in London. Dr. Cornwallis Hewitt, physician at St. George's Hospital in London, carried out a number of postmortems on victims, reporting (at approximately the same time as Trousseau and Bretonneau) the presence of "follicular ulcerations of the bowels," specifically in the Peyer's patches. Hewitt failed to recognize their significance.[37] In 1827 Dr. Richard Bright, a physician at Guy's Hospital in London, published his own observations of postmortems from the 1825–1826 outbreak. In addition to describing the fevers, Bright included illustrations and interpretations of his observations: "Whatever may be the primary nature of the febrile attack, there can be no doubt that early in the disease ... *almost always* [italics added], the intestinal canal is irritated, and that this irritation keeps up all the bad symptoms.... This vascularity is more generally connected with inflammation of the mucous glands, which often appear like the small-pox on the second or third day of eruption.... They scarcely seem to go into a state of true suppuration, but become distended with a yellow cheesy matter, and slough off; or sometimes ulceration takes place upon their points externally, without any collection of yellow matter being perceptible."[38] Budd pointed out the significance of the "almost always" in Bright's description. While Bright unquestionably had observed in some patients the ulceration which resulted from typhoid, other lesions found in other victims were not typical of typhoid; rather, "fever" was the result of other causes.[39]

The September 1836 issue of the *Dublin Journal of Medical Science* contained two letters written by Dr. H.C. Lombard of Geneva to a Dr.

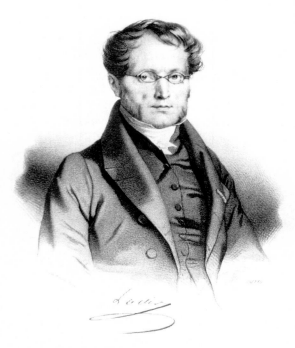

Pierre Charles Alexandre Louis (1787–1872), French physician noted for his application of statistical analysis in study of disease. Louis was the first to propose the name typhoid fever in identification of that disease (courtesy National Library of Medicine).

Robert Graves, describing his observations and conclusions about the relationship between typhus fever, which was present in Britain, and dothienenteritis in France and elsewhere on the European continent. Lombard had studied the latter disease during the previous six years, and in essentially all cases in France observed the presence of lesions on the Peyer's patches of victims. While visiting Glasgow and Dublin earlier in 1836, Lombard had the opportunity to carry out postmortem examinations of several victims of similar fevers. Despite the symptoms of their final illness being similar to those exhibited by the French victims, he found the characteristic lesions previously observed in the Peyer's patches to be absent. Lombard later visited fever hospitals in several cities in England where he received secondhand accounts of similar postmortem examinations. He was told that such ulcerations were sometimes present, but often not. In the first of the letters, Lombard described those findings:

> You are well aware of the different views entertained in France and England concerning this important subject; on the one hand the French pathologists and most recent writers, such as Louis, have described the continued fever named typhus [dothienenteritis], as being always attended by a certain pathological state of the intestinal canal, which begins with swelling and enlargement of the groups of follicular glands, situated in the lower third of the ileum, and forming the oval patches termed *glandulae Peyerianae*. This process is according to them a constant attendant on typhus, and in fatal cases always ends in ulcerations of the mucous membrane. The English pathologists, on the other hand, have stated that although they do occasionally meet with the state of mucous membrane described by Louis, yet they do not consider it as being an essential ingredient of fever, and they maintain that fever of a continued and typhous character, is not necessarily connected with any particular morbid appearance or change in the intestinal canal.[40]

In the second of his letters to the journal, Lombard expressed his opinion: "I consider Ireland as the source of the continued typhous [*sic*] fever which prevails in Great Britain; it is there that it is generated, or rather constantly transmitted from one individual to another; your fever is what the French pathologists have called *typhus, typhus contagieux, fièvre des armées, fièvre des prisons* [contagious fever, army fever, jail fever].… You have two different fevers, one highly contagious, which I may call the *Irish typhus*, and in which the cephalic symptoms predominate, to the exclusion of abdominal alterations; the other which is sporadic, and most likely not so infectious, and in which the abdominal symptoms are more predominant, so much so that the follicular disease and consequent ulcerations are always to be found."[41] Thus, Lombard came very close to differentiating between two unique diseases, lacking only a more thorough analysis of the intestinal ulcerations as a defining feature in the respective illnesses.

It only remained for two Philadelphia physicians, William Gerhard and Casper W. Pennock, to conclusively prove that the typhus of Great Britain was identical to what was often referred to as jail, camp or ship fever and was a disease easily communicated between persons (through the vector of lice), while typhoid fever in France was a separate and unique disease, less easily transmitted directly between persons. An outbreak of fever which had taken place during the spring and summer of 1836 in

Philadelphia was investigated by the two physicians, each of whom had previously had experience studying the enteric fever present in France. Both Gerhard and Pennock, as noted earlier, had been students of Louis. In two articles they published in 1837, the significant differences between the two diseases were highlighted. In particular, they pointed out that the lesions invariably found on the Peyer's patches in typhoid victims were never present in cases of typhus. Other differences included the forms of rash found in the two illnesses—small, petechial spots in the case of typhus, larger rose-colored rashes in cases of typhoid:

1. Dothinenteritis is usually a sporadic disease, although it sometimes appears as a widespread epidemic. In the latter case the symptoms are so well marked, that these are never doubtful, except in a few of the earliest examples. Now, typhus is very rarely sporadic, and if scattering cases do occur, they are generally connected with an epidemic and follow it, as scattering cases of the cholera were observed for a time after the great epidemic of 1832.

2. Typhus is evidently very contagious; in the epidemic of 1836 it was quite as contagious as smallpox.... Dothinenteritis is certainly not contagious under ordinary circumstances, although in some epidemics we have strong reason to believe that it becomes so.

3. The initial symptoms of the two affections chiefly differ in the greater stupor, dullness and prostration of typhus, which are in strong contrast to the moderate cephalalgia and disturbance of the senses of dothinenteritis....

When the disease [dothinenteritis] is completely formed, the characters on which the distinctions between the two forms of fever rest, are: 1. The suffusion of the eyes, which occurs in every case, or nearly every case of typhous fever, with the dusky-red aspect of the countenance. 2. The extreme stupor and inactivity of the mind even when positive delirium does not exist. 3. We also observe in typhus no constant abdominal symptom,

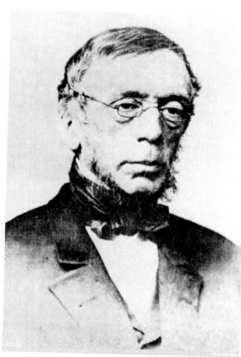

William Gerhard (1809–1872), American physician and among the first to suggest typhoid fever was a unique disease (courtesy Wellcome Library, London).

and at first merely dullness on percussion and feebleness of respiration at the posterior surface of the lungs. 4. If to these symptoms be added the peculiar eruption of petechiae, which is scarcely ever absent … there remains hardly a possibility of error. In the typhoid fever we consider as distinctive characters, the prostration, the somnolence, the slow development of nervous symptoms, which are not so strongly marked as in typhus. The abdominal symptoms are tympanitis, pains in the abdomen, and diarrhea. The sibilant rhonchus is heard in the chest; and, lastly, there is an eruption of rose-coloured papulae and sudamina [rash] upon the skin.[42]

The accumulation of evidence, particularly that reported by Gerhard and Pennock, was sufficient to convince most physicians, including Louis, of the unique nature of the two diseases. During the years immediately following their 1837 report, others confirmed their observations while adding little of substance that was new. Lemuel Shattuck, a Boston statistician, politician and founder of the American Statistical Association (1839), noted the differences in the epidemiological characteristics of the two diseases while compiling vital statistics for the city. Though Shattuck had carried out committee work with the American Medical Association on applications of vital statistics, he was not a trained physician. And while most physicians acknowledged the difference, it was not universal. Some still remained skeptical about whether typhus and typhoid were really two entirely different illnesses.

It was Sir William Jenner who finally completed the comparison of typhus and typhoid fever. Jenner,

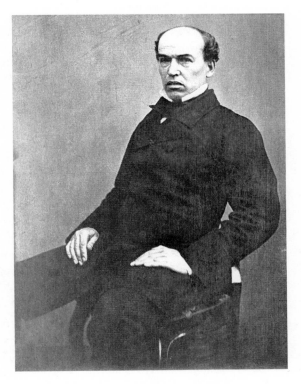

Sir William Jenner (1815–1898), British physician whose comparison of the enteric fevers led to the definitive differentiation of typhoid and typhus. Jenner became the primary physician for Queen Victoria during the illness and subsequent death of the Prince Consort, Albert (courtesy Wellcome Library, London).

who would later serve as physician to Queen Victoria and Albert, the Prince Consort (see Chapter 6), carried out an analysis of nearly 1,000 patients under the care of Dr. Alexander Tweedie at the London Fever Hospital between 1849 and 1851. Jenner's descriptions demonstrated to nearly all remaining skeptics the distinctiveness of the two fevers. The results, read in December 1849 before a British surgical society, were first published in the *Monthly Journal,* then independently as a treatise. Jenner began by acknowledging that the separate nature of the diseases alleged by Gerhard, Shattuck and others was not universally accepted:

> Whether the primary affection is identical in typhus and typhoid fevers is the problem to be solved. Are the differences allowed to exist between them due simply to individual peculiarities, atmospheric differences, epidemic constitutions, or hygienic conditions, giving rise to local complications in the one which are absent in the other, and to variations in the symptoms as a consequence of these local complications? Or are they distinct diseases, as are scarlet fever and smallpox?—distinct as to their primary or exciting cause, their essential symptoms, and their anatomical lesions. It may be as well, before proceeding further, to anticipate a little, and to state that the conclusion necessarily drawn from the analysis about to be submitted to the reader of sixty-six fatal cases of the fever, is in opposition to the opinion of the principal writers on the subject of continued fever in this country. With few exceptions, British physicians have labored to prove that typhoid and typhus fevers are identical.[43]

Jenner began by dividing the sixty-six fatal cases into two groups on the basis of the postmortem examination: those in which lesions in the Peyer's patches were readily visible (23 victims), and those in which those glands appeared healthy (43 victims). Applying 21st century vernacular to Jenner's work, victims in each group were compared in order to determine whether anything other than superficial variables were present. The mean height of men was approximately the same in each group, as was the mean height of women. There was some age difference—mean age for men in the typhus group was approximately 42 years, and for the men in the typhoid group it was approximately 22 years. All members of each group had appeared healthy prior to their illness. Thus, there were no significant variables which might account for two forms of the same illness, as alleged by some British physicians.

Jenner supported his viewpoint by comparing a wide range of symptoms associated with each form of the fevers: onset and duration, as far as could be determined, and physical changes such as headache, diarrhea, the appearance of spots or a rash, and, in particular, abdominal pain. These symptoms were then correlated with the presence or absence of intestinal lesions. Jenner used as an analogy the differences between smallpox and scarlet fever, applying those differences in his argument pertaining to typhus and typhoid (with Jenner's comparison of typhus and typhoid included in parentheses):

> At the commencement of this analysis I proposed to examine whether typhoid fever and typhus fever differed from each other in the same way as small-pox and scarlet fever differed from each other; and, for the purpose of comparison, I laid down certain grounds, as those on which we founded our belief in the non-identity of the two last-named diseases. These grounds were:—
>
> 1st, In the vast majority of cases the general symptoms differ—i.e., of small-pox and scarlet fever. (This holds equally true with respect to the general symptoms of typhoid and typhus fevers.)
>
> 2d, The eruptions, the diagnostic characters, *if present*, are never identical—i.e., in small-pox and scarlet fever. (The particulars detailed in the foregoing papers prove that this is as true of the eruptions of typhoid and typhus fever, as of those of small-pox and scarlet fever.)
>
> 3d, The anatomical character of small-pox is never seen in scarlet fever. (Just in same way the anatomical character of typhoid fever—i.e., lesion of Peyer's patches and the mesenteric glands—is never seen in typhus fever.)
>
> 4th, Both—i.e., small-pox and scarlet fever—being contagious diseases, the one by no combination of peculiarities, atmospheric variations, epidemic constitutions, or hygienic conditions, can give rise to the other. (I have here not attempted to determine how far this holds true with respect to typhoid and typhus fevers; but I have considered it in a paper read before the Medico-Chirurgical Society of London, December 1849 [alluded to above], the contents of which I may anticipate so far as to state, that to my mind the origin of the two diseases from distinct specific causes, is as clearly proved as that scarlet fever and small-pox arise from distinct specific causes.)
>
> 5th, The epidemic constitution, favourable to the origin, spread, or peculiarity in form or severity of either—i.e., small-pox and scarlet fever—has no influence over the other, excepting that which it exerts over disease in general. (The facts detailed in these papers prove that this holds as true of typhoid and typhus fevers as of small-pox and scarlet fever.)[44]

Jenner was even more assertive in the presentation before the Medico-Chirurgical Society the previous December: "I have ... expressed myself as if the specific cause respectively of typhoid fever, typhus fever, and relapsing fever, was an influence emanating from the bodies of those affected with either disease. With respect to the contagious nature of typhus fever, I know no one who entertains a doubt. If typhoid fever be contagious, it is infinitely less so than typhus fever. My experience leads me to regard it as contagious. Those who believe typhoid fever to be non-contagious while they admit the contagious nature of typhus fever, cannot for a moment doubt the difference in the specific causes of the diseases."[45]

After Jenner's analysis and conclusions, which ultimately received widespread acceptance even among most skeptics, one major question remained: how exactly did the patient contract the disease? During the 1850s and 1860s, the germ theory of disease was still a decade or more in the future. But inference built upon indirect evidence began to point to a fecal-oral method of transmission—more specifically through the ingestion of feces-contaminated water or food.

William Budd and the Fecal-Oral Connection

Born in 1811 to an English physician with a practice in North Tawton, William Budd grew up as one of ten sons and developed his interest in medicine as an apprentice to his father. Desiring to further his education in the medical field, in 1828 Budd made the first of what would ultimately be three visits to Paris in the course of his early career. There he had the opportunity to study internal medicine with the aforementioned François Broussais. Broussais at the time was one of the most influential of teachers, particularly in the area of physiological medicine, a viewpoint which included the use of leeches or emetics in treating disease. He believed that fever was the result of local inflammation and should be treated in that manner.[46] To Broussais, the lesions in the Peyer's patches represented this same sort of inflammation. In 1833 Budd traveled a second time to Paris, this time observing patients with Pierre Louis. Budd was significantly influenced by Louis's methods of observation, considering his work to be "admirable and elaborate."[47]

In 1838 Budd graduated with a medical degree from the University of Edinburgh, after which he became involved with the medical establishment in London through the colleagues of his brother George Budd as well as through serving at the naval hospital HMS *Dreadnaught*. Budd himself fortunately survived a case of typhoid fever while at the hospital. In the summer of 1839 he returned to North Tawton, a village of some 1,300 persons, in time to observe an epidemic of fever which broke out in July. Already familiar with typhoid fever as a result of his association with Louis and his own brush with the disease, Budd was convinced this was the identical disease. More specifically, he believed this was not the same disease as typhus fever.[48] That year the Provincial Medical and Surgical Association, a group which later became the British Medical Association, held an essay competition for the William Thackeray Prize on the topic of "the investigation of the sources of the common Continued Fevers of Great Britain and Ireland" and called for discussion of whether those diseases might be communicable.[49] Budd's summary of the North Tawton epidemic became the basis for his thesis in the essay that typhus and typhoid were unique diseases. Using specific examples, Budd summarized his argument:

> At first the people involved did not seem to have connections. However, the fourth case, a sawyer, removed to his home nine miles off, soon began to droop. Two days after his return home he was laid up with fever … [and] ten days after his death his two children were also laid up with fever and both had it severely. The widow remained well…. The case of the other sawyer (the sixth of the epidemic) who left the village when he felt the first symptoms of fever and went through the disease at his own home nearly nine miles off, is still more instructive. A friend who visited this man when he was at his worst, and was called upon to assist him in the bed … at the end of ten days was seized with rigor which was followed by typhoid fever of long duration…. This person now became a new source of contagion. Before he was convalescent, two of his children were laid up with fever, and also a brother, who lived at some distance, but who had repeatedly visited him.[50]

Budd's argument as to the contagious nature of the disease, as well as its unique identity, was admittedly weak: "That circumstances relating to the existence of contagious principles in latent form compel us to allow that these facts may possibly be explained on the supposition of contagion being the sole origin of fever: although it cannot be shown in our present state of knowledge, that this explanation will apply to all the circumstances of the case."[51] Budd left open the possibility that there might be other explanations for the outbreak.

In 1841 or 1842 Budd moved to Bristol, where he served as a physician at St. Peter's Hospital, housed in a fifteenth-century mansion, and the Bristol Royal Infirmary.[52] Two events led Budd to the conclusion that the source of typhoid might be a contaminated water supply. In 1847, while visiting a patient in nearby Clifton, he learned that an epidemic of typhoid had broken out in 13 of the 34 households in the Richmond Terrace portion of the town. In attempting to trace the possible source for the 13 affected households, Budd determined the only common denominator was a well they shared. The 21 unaffected households all obtained their water from a different source.[53] The second event was associated with a different disease: cholera. In 1849 John Snow determined the likely source of a cholera outbreak in London was a contaminated water supply. Budd became convinced that a possible source of typhoid might also be a contaminated water supply.

When he was appointed health officer in Bristol in 1849, one of his actions was to ensure a sanitary water supply.

Budd's investigation of other outbreaks during the 1850s convinced him that his original premise was correct, that the source of typhoid was sewage contamination of water supplies. In his 1873 work he summarized some of these examples:

> On February the 29th, 1864, I was summoned to the Convent of the Good Shepherd, at Arno's Court, near Bristol, to advise in a great emergency.... The structure, when completed, was divided into three principal segments. The community of Sisters, then 25 in number, lived in the old mansion; the next division was a reformatory for girls, of whom there were 126; the third was occupied by penitents, to the number of 34.... In March 1863, diarrhea appeared in the reformatory, and, in the course of two months, more than 50 of the girls were under medical treatment for it.
>
> But, unless the ailments here named belong to the self-propagating class, up to the date of the events about to be recorded no one of the recognised infections had ever attacked the inmates.... It is specially important to note, *that at no time, whether the drains were at their best or their worst, had typhoid fever ever appeared within the walls* [italics in original].
>
> The origin of this terrible outbreak was to the last degree clear. The disease was introduced into the convent in the preceding November, by a young girl who was admitted to the reformatory, *while actually laboring under it* ... the fever-stricken girl was admitted, the discharges were thrown down the infirmary cabinet, her clothes went with those of the other girls to the common wash-house, and were washed by the girls employed there. There was no idea of any precaution being necessary.

The outbreak was brought under control only after a disinfectant was added to the drain water.[54]

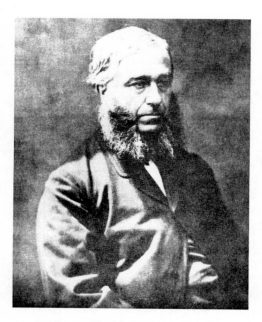

William Budd (1811–1880), British physician who confirmed the contagious nature of typhoid while describing the outbreaks in England during the 1860s and 1870s (courtesy Wellcome Library, London).

A second example Budd used to support his hypothesis concerned an outbreak in Frome during November 1863, which affected some 40 persons. The source of the outbreak was a "pauper" who was brought to Frome while convalescing from a case of typhoid. Shortly after her arrival, an epidemic of the disease broke out in the surrounding area. When sources of water which were in the vicinity of the drains or privies at the sites of the outbreak were closed, the epidemic faded out.[55] As Budd later wrote, "If it be certain that the intestinal discharges of this fever are the principal means of propagating the disease, it is no less certain that by subjecting the discharge on their issue from the body to the action of powerful disinfectants, they may be deprived of this property."[56] That is, if fecal discharges are disinfected, an epidemic will not take place.

Budd found the Thames River, which flowed through London, a particular source of contagion. That it was highly polluted from the effuse of 3 million citizens of the city was no surprise to anyone capable of breathing. The summer of 1858 served as a notable example. It was a time of unrest in the British colony of India. That, and the odors from the river, had a notable effect on the meeting of Parliament. A story in the newspaper so attested:

> For the first time in the history of man, the sewage of nearly three million people had been brought to seethe and ferment under a burning sun, in one vast open cloaca lying in their midst. The result we all know. Stench so foul, we may well believe, had never before ascended to pollute this lower air. Never before, at least, had a stink risen to the height of an historic event. For many weeks the atmosphere of Parliamentary Committee-rooms was only rendered barely tolerable by the suspension before every window, of blinds saturated with chloride of lime, and by the lavish use of this and other disinfectants. More than once, in spite of similar precautions, the law courts were suddenly broken up by an insupportable invasion of the noxious vapors from the river. The river steamers lost their accustomed traffic, and travelers pressed for time often made a circuit of many miles rather than cross one of the city bridges.... At home and abroad the state of the chief river was felt to be a national reproach. 'India is in Revolt and the Thames stinks' were the two great facts coupled together by a distinguished foreign writer, to mark the climax of a national humiliation. But more significant still of the magnitude of the nuisance was the fact that five million pounds were cheerfully voted to provide the means for its abatement [British Royal Commission on Sewage Disposal].[57]

Budd's conclusion was clear: "The great fact remains that sewers are the principal channels through which this fever is propagated, the proof from all sides is overwhelming that they are so not because of their being receptacles of decomposing organic matter, but solely due to their being depositories of the specific discharges of persons already infected."[58] A forceful and determined man, Budd was passionate about the means to prevent outbreaks of typhoid. His rules included the use of strong disinfectants like carbolic acid and chloride of lime, boiling potentially contaminated drinking water, and thoroughly sanitizing a patient's clothes and bed linens. In his view, the means to control or prevent such epidemics were relatively simple.

6

Of Princes and Presidents

I who felt, when in those blessed arms clasped and held tight in the sacred hours at night, when the world seemed only to be ourselves, that nothing could part us. I felt so very secure.—Victoria, Queen of England[1]

Victoria and Albert

In some respects Victoria was an accidental queen, the beneficiary of circumstances and tragedies in the royal line. Her grandfather was George III of American Revolutionary War fame. George III, who reigned until 1820, and his wife, Charlotte of Mecklenburg-Strelitz, had thirteen children, offspring which included seven males who would have been next in line for the throne. Upon George's death, the throne would pass to his son, the Prince of Wales and future George IV. Unlike the royal lineages in the rest of Europe, which passed only through a male line, the hereditary position of reigning monarch in England could subsequently pass from George IV either to his daughter, Princess Charlotte, or to his brothers in the order of their births.

Tragedy intervened. George and his wife, Caroline of Brunswick, had only that one child, Charlotte. However, Charlotte died in 1817 during a childbirth characterized by incompetent treatment by her physicians; the child was stillborn. George IV himself died in 1830.

The effects on the royal lineage would have done credit to a Shakespearean play. Next in line after George IV would normally have been his brother Frederick, Duke of York; but Frederick died in 1827, childless. William, Duke of Clarence, was next. Following the death of his brother in 1830, he became king, William IV. However, his marriage to Adelaide of Saxe-Meiningen did not produce an heir; the ten children with his mistress did not count. William IV died in 1837, and the throne would normally

69

have passed to his brother Edward, Duke of Kent. However, Edward had died in 1820, two years after his marriage to Victoire of Saxe-Coburg-Saalfeld. But they had one daughter, Alexandrina Victoria, born May 24, 1819, who would become queen following the death of William IV in 1837.[2]

Francis Albert Augustus Charles Emanuel—Albert, Prince Consort—was born August 26, 1819, at Schloss Rosenau near the town of Coburg in Bavaria, the second son of Ernest II, Duke of Saxe-Coburg-Saalfeld and Louise of Saxe-Gotha-Altenburg. Victoire, the future Queen Victoria's mother, was the sister of the Duke, Albert's father, meaning Victoria and Albert were actually cousins when they wed.

Almost from his birth, Albert's family groomed him as the potential prince consort for the throne of England. In many respects he grew into a perfect match for Victoria. Strikingly handsome, well-schooled, the latest in a long and proper bloodline, he also possessed a feature, almost unique among the males in the upper classes of the time and one of particular importance to Victoria. He was a virgin.[3]

The first meeting between Victoria and Albert took place in May 1836 in celebration of Victoria's seventeenth birthday. The two were still in their mid-teens and Victoria's uncle was on the throne. The meeting did not go particularly well, largely because Albert was simply not ready to prepare for matrimony, as "agreeable" as Victoria might have been in his eyes. As one biographer put it, "Their colt had been entered in a race before he was ready to run, but he still had excellent potential."[4]

On June 20, 1837, William IV died, and the throne passed to Victoria, his niece. She was aware that Albert would be among many potential suitors for her hand in marriage. But at the time, while admittedly fond of Albert, Victoria felt no particular attraction for her German cousin; the feeling was largely mutual. Once Victoria became queen things began to change, helped in part by catalysts in the form of her uncle King Leopold in Brussels and her mother as well. By early October 1839 Victoria agreed to at least "look over" Albert. When they again met early that month it was clear he was no longer the shy teenager Victoria had met earlier but had grown into a man. On October 14, using the proper protocol for their relative positions, she proposed. The wedding was held the following February (1840).

Victoria and Albert eventually had nine children, four sons and five daughters. The first, Victoria Adelaide Mary, Princess Royal, was born almost exactly nine months after the wedding. She later married Frederick III of Germany, and their son Wilhelm would become Kaiser Wilhelm II, the German ruler during the First World War. Victoria and Albert's second

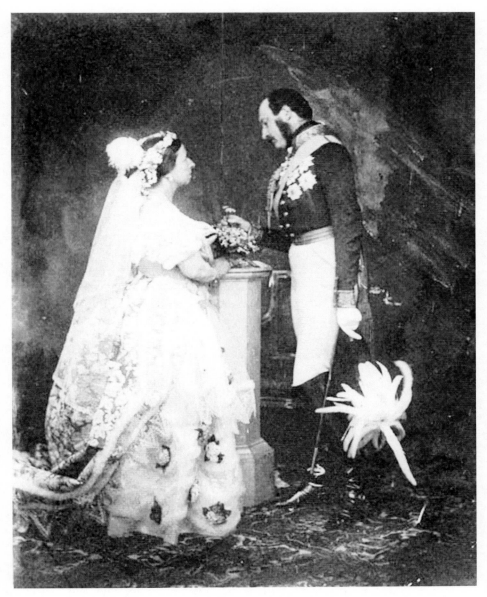

Queen Victoria and Albert, Prince Consort (1819–1861). First cousins, Victoria and Albert married in 1840. Though his powers were limited as Prince Consort, Albert instituted significant reforms in education and economic matters and played a significant role as an advisor for foreign policy. Victoria never fully recovered from her loss following his death from typhoid (courtesy Wellcome Library, London).

child and first son, Albert Edward, who was known as "Bertie," was born November 9, 1841, and would become King Edward VII upon Victoria's death some sixty years later. Their third child, Alice Maud Mary, born in 1843, married Louis IV, Grand Duke of Hesse. Alice and Louis's daughter Alexandra would marry Czar Nicholas II of Russia and would be murdered during the Russian Revolution. Thus three of Victoria's grandchildren, Edward VII's son George V, Kaiser Wilhelm and Alexandra, the czarina of Russia, were all first cousins.

To say Bertie would prove to be a challenge for his parents would be a mild understatement. Among those challenges would be his string of mistresses, both before and after his marriage to Princess Alexandra of Denmark. In fact, it was one of his liaisons which may indirectly have contributed to his father's death. During the summer of 1861 Bertie had attended a military camp at the Curragh in Ireland. That September on at least three occasions he had snuck out through a window for liaisons with a dance-hall girl and camp follower, Nellie Clifden. By November she had become a de facto mistress, even, according to sources, being smuggled into Windsor Castle for Bertie's birthday. Bertie later denied Clifden had been at his party; it does appear, however, that while Clifden was not, at least one other prostitute had been.[5]

The rumors of Bertie's behavior reached the Prince Consort shortly afterwards, and to say Albert was appalled would be understating his response. There was more than simply the activity of a young man at issue here, even though realistically an activity common within his social class. Clifden was already being known as the Princess of Wales, and the Prince Consort was (correctly) concerned that if she became pregnant, the Prince of Wales would be drawn into a scandal which might very well include blackmail. The father's first response was to send a letter admonishing his son for his behaviors "with a heavy heart, on a subject which has cost me the deepest pain I have yet felt in this life…. Albert regretted Bertie had found it acceptable "to thrust yourself into the hands of one of the most abject of the human species, to be by her initiated in the sacred mysteries of creation, which ought to remain shrouded in holy awe until touched by pure and undefiled hands."[6]

Exactly when Albert actually became ill is uncertain, but it was unquestionably some time before his November meeting with his son. Nevertheless, he was determined to carry out what he felt were his obligations as Victoria's husband as well as his duties as a father. On November 22 Albert traveled from Windsor to Sandhurst for an inspection of the newly completed buildings at the Staff College and Military Academy. Being late

November, the weather was miserable—cold and rainy—and Albert returned home wet and chilled, suffering from what he described as "rheumatism" as well as sleeplessness. On the 23rd he rode a special train to Madingley Hall near Cambridge to meet with Bertie with the intention of further addressing the son's relationship with Clifden, or at least to discuss his behavior in general. As on the previous day, the weather was cold, and in a heavy rain father and son spent several hours walking and discussing Bertie's behavior. It did not help that Bertie became lost, extending the time he and his father were in the elements. The Prince Consort returned home that night, again thoroughly wet and chilled. Victoria blamed his symptoms—depression, insomnia and even the "rheumatism"—on the stress of dealing with their son. It was equally likely they represented the developing stages of typhoid.

During the week which followed, Albert's symptoms only grew worse. Even though in hindsight it is clear Albert was feeling the effects of his illness, he was still able to walk over a parade ground at Eton on the 29th. Despite the day being warm for the season Albert was chilled and wore a heavy fur-lined coat. It was on the 30th November and the 1st of December that he carried out the last of his duties for the government, the revision of a note to be sent to the Lincoln administration over the *Trent* affair.

During the early months of the American Civil War, a Union ship, the *San Jacinto*, captured a British vessel, *Trent* and removed two Southern envoys who were traveling to England. The action had the potential to ignite a war between England and the United States. The initial note drafted by Lord Palmerston, the British prime minister, allowed for little maneuvering on the part of the American government. The revisions incorporated into the final draft by Prince Albert, and approved by the queen, allowed for face-saving measures and ultimately the resolution of an embarrassing diplomatic blunder.

That day, the 1st, Albert was clearly severely ill, with an increasing temperature, loss of appetite and chills, all signs of typhoid. Among the doctors now in attendance was William Jenner, by then considered among the most important medical consultants of his day (see below), as well as Sir James Clark, physician-in-ordinary to Queen Victoria in addition to his duties as Albert's physician. Clark was in the process of retiring by 1861, and the diagnosis and much of the treatment was delegated to Jenner.

By December 6 Jenner observed the presence of rose-colored spots on Albert's torso, and while confirming to Victoria that her husband was suffering from fever, he still held out hope for recovery. However, two days later Albert was delirious, failing to recognize even Victoria. The public was finally notified on the 11th of the Prince Consort's illness, and Albert himself acknowledged that he was likely dying. Bertie was finally summoned to his father's bedside—the call had been delayed on the orders of Victoria in hopes Albert would recover, and to prevent her son's exposure to the illness—on the 13th. It was only then the Prince of Wales learned how sick his father actually was.[7] The end came at 10:45 p.m. on the 14th, with Victoria holding his hand: "Oh, this is death! I know it. I have seen it before."[8]

Once Albert was infected there was, of course, little the doctors could do beyond providing opium for comfort and perhaps help alleviate the diarrhea. Four were in attendance with the Prince Consort at various times during his illness: Clark, Jenner, Thomas Watson and Henry Holland. Standard treatment of the time often involved bleeding, but Albert at least was spared that.

An explanation was provided to the public, addressing both lack of notification as well as the course of the illness itself:

The insidious character of this disease is always opposed to any early and decisive diagnosis of its precise character. Moreover, its first symptoms are common to various mild forms of febrile disorder.... If the disease by which the Prince Consort fell was by no means of that ambiguous and usually innocent character which popular report has assigned to it, no doubt from misinterpretation of the necessary official reticence of the earlier bulletins, so also it should be observed that the illness was of longer duration than at first appeared. The Prince Consort had been attacked at least a fortnight before the fatal termination. On Sunday week he was unable to attend Divine service, a duty ever held as of paramount importance in his well-balanced mind. On the Monday following Dr. Jenner was summoned, and from that time the Prince was under continuous medical advice. It is perhaps commonly thought that, as a man of middle age, well-nourished, and of course highly cared for in all material wants, the Prince might have been less than usually liable to fall a victim to low fever of this kind. But the opposite series of relations may always be predicted in typhoid fever. This is a disease which has invariably proved far more fatal to sufferers of the upper class and of middle period of life than to patients of the poorer kind. The unhappy issue must therefore be regarded as a source of deep lamentation rather than of surprise. There is nothing in the known course of the disease during the last week of the attack to take it out of the ordinary character of typhoid fever. The immediate cause of death is believed to have been congestion of the lungs.... The congestion was, of course, hypostatic or gravitative [accumulation of blood], and such as occurs in the last stages of weakness of the circulation. On the other hand, there was enough of suddenness in the immediate termination of the disease to raise the question whether it might not have been due to ulcerative perforation of the bowel, a well-known complication of typhoid fever.[9]

The doctors acknowledged the diagnosis had been made late, likely for a reason. In the context of the time, a diagnosis of "fever" would have quickly been interpreted as typhoid fever by the family. Clark and Jenner were afraid this would have sent Victoria into hysterics, and as well affected the morale of the patient.[10] To repeat, there was little beyond palliative treatment the doctors could have done anyway.

Progress of Albert's Final Illness[11]

Date	Symptoms	Comments
November 22	Felt "horribly ill"	Cold, rainy day; Albert soaked: "*entsetzlicher regen*, a drenching rain"
November 23		Walked with Bertie in the cold rain
November 24–28	"Unwell," loss of appetite; insomnia; likely feverish	Returned to Windsor so weak his physician (Dr. William Jenner) stayed the night; Victoria reported Albert as "rheumatic" (aching?)
November 29–30	Chills and fever	Chills such that Albert wore fur-lined coat; walked on parade grounds
December 1	Fever; chills while sweating "profusely"; vomiting; loss of appetite; insomnia	Still able to dress and walk; family read to him; redrafted note to President Lincoln over *Trent* affair
December 2		Albert indicated he "had no fever"; likely just not in the diagnosis yet; among attending physicians was Dr. Jenner
December 3–4		Victoria indicated his illness was influenza
December 5–6	Observation of rash of spots on Albert's body; fever	Advised that Albert should remain in bed
December 7–8	Delirious; increasingly failed to recognize Victoria; irritable; rash developed on stomach and abdomen; tongue appeared dry and "furry"	Still able to move from room to room; asked to hear music, so Alice played German songs; moved to Blue Room; Albert acknowledged he might be dying.
December 9–11	Delirious; by the 10th too weak to dress	Sir Henry Holland and Dr. Thomas Watson now in attendance; bulletins released to public. On the 10th able to briefly sit up and drink tea; Victoria found him again sitting up on the 11th. The death of his cousin King

Date	Symptoms	Comments
		Pedro V of Portugal from typhoid, days before, was present in his mind, leading to his belief he would not recover.
December 12	In pain; increasingly delirious; coughed up mucous; chills; rapid breathing	Albert given opium and ether to sleep and relieve pain; soup and brown bread to eat; brandy
December 13	Breathing increasingly more rapid; skin took on a dusky hue	Given brandy; Victoria able to briefly take a break and go for a walk.
December 14	Died just prior to 11 p.m.	

These early years of Victoria and Albert's reign were still a decade or more before the development of the Germ Theory of Disease. Nevertheless the Prince Consort had been a strong proponent of sanitation in promoting health, which included understanding the need for clean water and proper drainage throughout the country. Even in the context of the twenty-first century Albert would have been considered "fastidiously clean," a "sanitarian"—an advocate of the importance of public health in the general population. Frequent exercise in fresh air and proper eating and drinking habits were components of his lifestyle. The residences he designed at Osborne and Balmoral included "state-of-the-art" facilities—toilets, baths and showers.[12]

So the question which remains here was how Albert was exposed to the disease. There is no shortage of possibilities. While his newer homes had modern—for the time—sewage systems, those sites he encountered elsewhere were no doubt lacking in equivalent facilities. One cannot rule out the possibility he may have even been exposed in the very place where he later died: Windsor Castle. The town of Windsor had experienced an outbreak of typhoid fever only two years earlier, the origin of which had been determined by Charles Murchison to be associated with improper drainage.[13] However, Murchison studied the plans, which disclosed the drainage system associated with both Windsor Castle and the surrounding town drained sewage from the castle directly into the Thames River. This was not the situation as it pertained to the Royal Mews, which were separated from the castle only by a roadway. That half of the Mews, which benefited from the castle drainage, was disease free, while the royal servants in the remaining portion, which was subjected to sewage contamination, suffered thirty cases of typhoid, including three deaths.[14] Albert may also

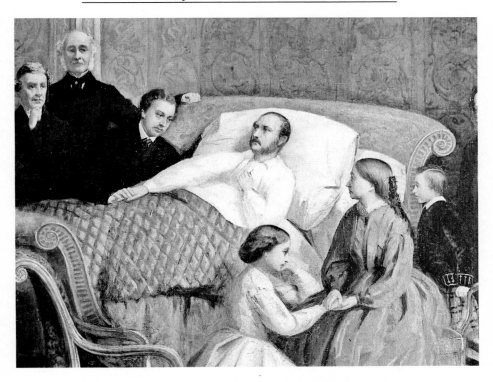

The Last Moments of Prince Albert, lithograph by W.I. Walton. Queen Victoria and William Jenner are among those depicted at his bedside. The queen is seated at right, holding the hand of a child; Jenner is the tall, bald man on the left (courtesy Wellcome Library, London).

have been exposed during his travels the previous month (November) to places such as Cambridge or South Kensington; the variable length of the incubation period creates a challenge when trying to narrow down the possible choices. Nor was Albert the only contemporary monarch who contracted the disease during these months. Earlier in that same month of November during which Albert had been exposed, both twenty-five year-old King Pedro (Peter) V of Portugal and his younger brother Ferdinand died of the same disease. (Pedro and Ferdinand were closely related to Victoria and Albert; their father, Ferdinand Coburg-Kohary was a first cousin.)

It should be noted that alternative causes of Albert's fatal illness have been suggested: stomach cancer and even Crohn's disease.[15] Albert reportedly suffered from repeated bouts of gum inflammation, the source of which can be fumes associated with over-secretion of stomach acid. Such overproduction of hydrochloric acid can result in peptic ulcers and even carcinoma of the stomach. Albert's family history included the fact that his mother died from the disease at the age of thirty. But given the symptoms of the Prince Consort's final illness and the almost endemic presence of typhoid, it appears highly unlikely his death had been the result of stomach cancer. Nor would the rash described by William Jenner be likely in the case of Crohn's disease. So while one cannot rule out the possibilities of ulcerative colitis or even Crohn's as contributing factors to Albert's ongoing health problems, it is highly unlikely they would account for his final illness. The fact was that even in the years after Albert's death British royalty was not always protected from the danger of contaminated sewage; it was often the lifestyle associated with royalty itself which placed the person at greater risk:

Czar Nicholas' prostration by typhoid fever (followed so quickly after the death of her [Victoria's] grandson, Prince Christian Victor of Schleswig-Holstein, from the same malady [October 1900]), serves to call attention to the havoc which this particular disease has played in the family of England's aged sovereign. Her husband succumbed thereto forty years ago; the Prince of Wales was laid low by it in 1870 and brought to the brink of the grave [see below]. His younger son, the Duke of York, had his constitution permanently impaired by an attack of typhoid, while his elder brother, Edward, Duke of Clarence [1892]; the Queen's son-in-law, Prince Henry of Battenberg [1896], the Kaiser's brother Sigismund [1866], as well as several other members of Queen Victoria's family circle have been carried off thereby.... No matter what the modern luxuries and conveniences with which they have been equipped they retain the foundations of bygone ages, when sewerage, as now understood and applied, was virtually unknown; there are few royal palaces in existence, the subsoil of which is absolutely reeking with the sewage of centuries.

To give an idea of the extent to which this prevails, it may be mentioned that when, after the attack of typhoid to which the Duke of Clarence succumbed, and which inflicted such injury to the health of the Duke of York, Marlborough House, the town residence of the Prince of Wales and of his family, was subjected to a searching investigation. It was discovered that this palace, built by the first Duchess of Marlborough, barely two centuries ago, was resting, so to speak, on a swamp of sewage into which the subsoil had been converted through defective drainage.

Two years previously Buckingham Palace, the town residence of the Queen, a building even still less old than Marlborough House, was found to be in a similar position, matters being aggravated in that case by the fact that a huge metropolitan sewer, constructed more than one hundred years ago of brick, and serving the huge St. George's Hospital in the same district, ran right underneath the palace within a few feet of the basement, and, owing to faulty construction, was leaking in every direction.... Windsor Castle ... would be far worse were it not for the fact that it is perched upon an eminence, while the royal palaces at Madrid, Stockholm, the winter palace at St. Petersburg, the older portions of the Haufburg, Vienna, the royal palaces at Turin, Florence, and Naples are all simply germ beds of typhoid fever.[16]

Ten years after the death of the Prince Consort, Bertie, the Prince of Wales, contracted the same fever following his stay at Londesborough Lodge in the town of Scarborough during late October and early November 1871. The prince and his (by then) wife, Alexandra (Alix), were guests of Lord Londesborough along with some two dozen others for a week of grouse shooting. By November 9, the prince's thirtieth birthday, he began to complain of being chilled. Nevertheless, he traveled through a wicked gale to Buckinghamshire for recreational shooting, but he quickly became too ill to continue. Within several days the symptoms included fever and a rose-colored rash. His personal physician, Dr. William Gull, was called, and he diagnosed the illness as typhoid fever.

The prince's illness continued to increase in its severity, now with the inclusion of diarrhea and vomiting in addition to the aforementioned symptoms. His temperature peaked during mid–December with a fever of over 104°, and some newspapers even compared the prince's critical state with that of his father's ten years earlier. For a time he was even unable to recognize either his mother, Victoria, or his wife, Alix; his delirium included denial she was even his wife. At one point during what the prince's doctors thought was a death watch, William Jenner commented to Gull, "If he lives until Her Majesty [Victoria] comes I shall be satisfied." Gull replied, "That will not satisfy me."[17]

Recovery began about the 14th of December, the anniversary of Prince Albert's death. With the help of both Jenner and the prince's own personal physician, Dr. Gull (neither of whom prescribed the contemporary medicines, which might have even killed the prince), Bertie began to regain his strength. Restoration of Bertie's health was aided in no small part by his strong and youthful constitution as well as the care provided by both his wife and mother; the prince completely recovered after weeks of recuperation. Gull was awarded a baronetcy.[18]

An investigation by the Lancet Sanitary Commission was carried out to determine the source of the prince's illness. Londesborough Lodge was in a low-lying area, "at the summit of a great length of sewer, and no openings whatever are provided for the escape of gas or the relief of any pressure":

Furthermore, all the drains are unfortunately placed—the main ones in the centre of the building, and the branches running from the circumference to the centre underneath the floors. None of the soil-pipes open on the roof, and even the surface water-drains are all carefully trapped. The drains are thus placed in positions where they cannot be inspected, and where the least flaw will produce the greatest mischief. With such evidence as to the effect of the tide—with the probability that the rat found under the floor had escaped from the drain at some undiscovered point—with the additional draft produced by numerous fires and many gas-lights in a house with closed doors and windows, and with the defective watercloset pan—it seems impossible to doubt that the air of Londesborough Lodge was really tainted. There might be but little smell.[19]

The prince was not the only resident or guest to have been taken ill during this period. Among the victims of what was almost certainly typhoid were the Earl of Chesterfield, who occupied the state rooms following the departure of the prince and whose death from the illness was announced on December 1, the Duchess of Manchester, and even Lord Londesborough himself.[20] The commission proposed two possibilities for the source of the prince's illness:

> Some parts of the pheasant feeding grounds are rendered dangerous by the practice of hanging up carrion for the growth of the "gentles" on which the pheasants are fed. We have not thought it necessary to investigate this suggestion. There can be no offensive carrion at this time of year, and it is improbable that any offensive matters would have remained since the summer.
>
> The second is, that His Royal Highness might have been poisoned as he rode by a manure yard on the Seamer-road, the stench from which is certainly abominable. The Duke of Baeufort writes to say that the stench made him feel very sick, and that it made one of his servants ill. The place is no doubt a dangerous nuisance.... Fermentation rapidly begins, and the effluvia are offensive beyond description.... It is significant that this place is at the head of the valley sewer, into which Londesborough Lodge is drained.... We have, however, great difficulty in believing that a short exposure to this influence would give rise to typhoid fever. It is really wonderful how much the human frame will bear with impunity whilst under the influence of free exercise and ventilation in the open air. No matter how dangerous the stink, the effect is at once destroyed by a few inspirations of the rapidly moving air. It is within the walls, and especially in the night, that noxious effluvia exert their greatest influence, and it is just then that the system is least able to resist their force. We cannot therefore associate the origin of His Royal Highness's complaint with the casual inhalation of air from a possibly infected muckheap, nor, indeed, with the mere possibility that he has unwittingly been in the neighborhood of a person laboring under typhoid fever. Naturally of a strong constitution, His Royal Highness would resist for the longest possible duration the influence of any morbific poison, and the dose must have been strong and continuously taken to produce so grave a malady.[21]

Though they ultimately ruled it out, the commission clearly considered a pythogenic source for the disease, the effluvia or emanations of a fermentative process originating from the manure, rather than contamination of a water source from sewage. Again, this is no surprise, given the contemporary understanding of any role played by micro-organisms.

Sir William Jenner (1815–1898)

Sir William Jenner had a long and distinguished career in medicine and was known most notably as a primary physician to the royal family and for his role in firmly establishing the "non-identity" of typhus fever (jail fever) and typhoid fever in 1849. Jenner was born at Chatham on January 30, 1815, the fourth son of innkeepers John and Elizabeth Jenner. His medical education was carried out at University College, London, and following an apprenticeship in Marylebone he was awarded diplomas as Member Royal College of Surgeons of England (MRCS) and Licentiate of the Society of Apothecaries (LSA) London in 1837. He received his medical degree in 1844 from the University of London. Among his early medical appointments was that of the staff of the Royal Maternity Charity.

In the years immediately following the awarding of the degree, Jenner exchanged his general practice for that of medical consultant. It was during this period that he carried out the study which established the differentiation of typhus and typhoid fever (see below). In 1849 he was appointed to the position of professor of pathological anatomy at University College as well as assistant physician at the associated University College hospital. Five years later he was promoted to physician, ultimately becoming head of a new department for study of diseases of the skin. Jenner was honored with appointment to several important positions during these years, including physician to the London Fever Hospital, where he served from 1853 to 1861, physician to the Hospital for Sick Children, 1852 to 1862, and professor of the principles and practice of medicine at University College.

It was Jenner's study of patients admitted to the London Fever Hospital between January 1847 and February 1849 that laid the groundwork for the recognition of his medical talents. Work establishing the uniqueness of typhus and typhoid fever had been carried out by a number of physicians during the previous decade, including Pierre Louis in France, where typhoid fever had been endemic (1830s), William Gerhard and Casper Pennock in the United States (1837), and Drs. H.C. Barlow and Alexander Stewart (1840) in England. In fact, noted medical pioneer William Osler had commented on Gerhard's work as "the first in any language to give a full and satisfactory account of the clinical and anatomical distinctions that were later recognized and accepted."[22]

However, many people still were unconvinced and continued to believe that rather than being distinct diseases, typhus and typhoid fever represented varieties of the same disease. Certainly some of the more obvious symptoms, including a high fever and accompanying rash, were common to both diseases. Jenner's study, "On the Identity or Non-Identity of the Specific Cause of Typhoid, Typhus and Relapsing Fever," first published in 1849 and again the following year, analyzed both those symptoms the illnesses appeared to have in common as well as characteristics such as the intestinal lesions found in typhoid.[23] His conclusion, which ultimately gained widespread acceptance, was that these are distinct diseases. A more complete description of the specifics of Jenner's study is found elsewhere in this book.

In 1861, Dr. William Baly, one of Queen Victoria's physicians, died, and Jenner was appointed to the position of Physician Extraordinary and the following year to the more exalted position as Physician in Ordinary to Victoria, a position he would retain for a quarter century. It was during this period that Jenner was in attendance during the illness and death of the Prince Consort. In 1871 the Prince of Wales, the future King Edward VII, contracted the same disease which had killed his father; but with the medical assistance of Jenner, he was able to recover.

Jenner's honors continued for the remaining decades of his life. In 1868 he received a baronetcy, among the highest of the heritage honors and which entitled him to the designation of "Sir." In 1872 he became a Knight Commander of the Bath, and in 1889 to Grand Cross. In 1881 he was elected by his peers to the presidency of the Royal College of Physicians and was reelected another six times. He served as well in the presidency of several other professional societies.

Jenner's teaching in the clinical area was considered far advanced for the time. It was common for him to question his students "at the bedside, and lead them to observe for themselves. Errors of observation he sought to have corrected on the spot, and when the facts had been elicited he discussed their interpretation, usually expressing his own opinion with great distinctness, and occasionally giving utterance to some telling phrase which stuck in the memory.... It is certainly true that the clinical fact which Jenner sought to teach was thus indelibly impressed on the mind of the student.... "That is the opinion that I have come to from my observation; you must test it for yourself by your own observations!"[24]

Jenner's later years were marked by declining health. Upon his death in 1898 Queen Victoria expressed her feelings over the loss of more than just her physician: "The Queen received yesterday with much regret the news of the death of Sir William Jenner, who had been Her Majesty's physician for upwards of thirty years, and who only retired from the Queen's service in 1893, owing to failing health. He was not only a most able physician, but a true and devoted friend of Her Majesty's, who deeply mourns his loss."[25]

Prince Albert was not the only well-known political figure during that era to have succumbed to typhoid. Though the evidence is not entirely definitive, it is possible that one, and perhaps two, of the American presidents became infected and died while in office during the mid–19th century from what some have diagnosed as a typhoid infection: William Henry Harrison, 9th president of the United States (1841), and Zachary Taylor, 12th president of the United States (1849–1850). James Knox Polk, 11th president of the United States (1845–1849), died three months after leaving office from a gastrointestinal ailment, almost certainly cholera in this case. At least three other presidents, Grover Cleveland, William Howard Taft and Franklin Roosevelt, likely contracted typhoid during their youth or as young adults but recovered.

As has been discussed previously, the term gastrointestinal illness encompasses a wide range of possible ailments, from dysentery to cholera and, of course, enteric fevers. In the 1850s and 1860s, decades before the germ theory of disease was developed, the concept of an etiological agent was largely unknown. Therefore, one can only attempt to diagnose the ailments which killed the two presidents based upon contemporary descriptions of symptoms, much as we did in an earlier chapter addressing both the Plague of Athens and Alexander the Great's final illness. President Taylor's death in particular has become a source of controversy because of its alleged impact on the slavery issue.

William Henry Harrison (1773–1841)

William Henry Harrison is often the subject of presidential trivia: Which president had the shortest term in office, and which grandfather and grandson pair were presidents? Harrison died barely one month after his inauguration, and President Benjamin Harrison, the 23rd president, was his grandson.

Harrison was born February 9, 1773, into a large (eleven children) and wealthy Virginia family who were members of what has been referred to as the "planter aristocracy." His future grandson was only one of several family members who had an impact on American history. His father, Benjamin Harrison, was among the signers of the Declaration of Independence in 1776 as well as being a member of the Continental Congress and later governor of Virginia. A brother, Carter Harrison, served in the House of Representatives. After an education at Hampden-Sidney College William began the study of medicine. However, following the death of his father, he enlisted in the military in 1791, serving as aide-de-camp to General "Mad" Anthony Wayne, participating in the Battle of Fallen Timbers in Ohio in 1794, which effectively secured that region of the Northwest Territory for the nascent United States.

Harrison resigned from the army several years later and was subsequently appointed by President John Adams as governor of the Indiana Territory, serving from 1801 to 1812. Harrison achieved national fame when in 1811 he led an expedition against a consortium of Native American tribes in the territory, defeating them in a battle along the Tippecanoe River near Lafayette and northwest of present-day Indianapolis. Harrison served with distinction throughout the War of 1812, later building on his fame in holding a variety of state and national political offices. In 1840, under the banner of "Tippecanoe and [John] Tyler too" as the candidate for the Whig Party, he soundly defeated Martin Van Buren in the presidential election.

Harrison was inaugurated March 4, 1841, delivering the longest inaugural address in American presidential history, some 8,445 words, in wet freezing weather. He failed to dress accordingly, wearing neither hat nor coat nor gloves. History records that he caught a severe cold which developed into pneumonia, resulting in his death a month later.

Recently, Philip Mackowiak, professor in the Department of Medicine at the University of Maryland Medical School, has proposed an alternate explanation for Harrison's death: typhoid fever, with likely septic shock a contributing factor. The president may very well have contracted pneumonia, though even here there is some dispute, but this was not likely to have been the initial illness which ultimately ended his life.

Date	Symptoms and Complaints	Comments
March 26	Following "several days of anxiety and fatigue" he contacted his physician, Dr. Thomas Miller.	Harrison attributed his symptoms to the "intense physical and mental pressures" associated with the inauguration and his duties as president. The president had treated himself with an undisclosed medicine; Miller advised bed rest.

Date	Symptoms and Complaints	Comments
March 27	Miller again summoned (1:00 p.m.), because of chills. Mustard plaster was applied to the stomach while Harrison was given a warm drink containing diaphoretic draught (tartar emetic: antimony potassium tartrate) with *spiritus Mindereri* (acetate of ammonia). Harrison constipated, so given *Mars Hydrarg* (Hydrangea extract sometimes used to dissolve stones) (mercury) and *Etract. Colocynth Comp*, a laxative. Complained of pain over right eye.	The president told Miller that he had arisen about 4:00 a.m. and had taken a walk around the grounds. Severe chills had appeared while meeting with his cabinet about 90 minutes earlier than when the doctor was called. By 5:00 p.m. felt much improved. Skin was "warm and moist," while pulse was a relatively normal 75.
March 28	After midnight, complained pain over right eye was more severe as well as pain on right side. Miller ordered enema, mustard plaster and Seidlitz powder (tartaric acid/sodium bicarbonate/potassium tartrate) laxative. Given additional *Mars Hydrarg* along with *Pulvus Rhei* (rhubarb, ginger, magnesium oxide) laxative and camphor. Chills returned about noon; requested opium be applied to right side. At 3:00 a blistering preparation applied, as well as ingestion of laudanum and laxative. Later given 5 drops of calomel (mercury chloride) and laudanum.	Discomfort initially eased by morning with pain resolved late morning. About 11:30 became restless, with nausea that afternoon. By midafternoon his skin became warm with "hurried" breathing and flushing. Miller diagnosed possible pneumonia in right lung as well as liver congestion. The pain over the right eye was attributed to neuralgia. The opium allowed Harrison to sleep. Dr. Frederick May called in as a consultant by Miller, and who recommended the current treatment be continued.
March 29	Harrison received 2 more laxative pills and calomel. Later Miller provided Dover's powder (ipecac and opium), and castor oil for the constipation. Dark	Pulse 80 and "soft." At 2:00 p.m. began breathing heavily, with a dry cough. Pulse increased to 90 over the course of the day. The president consumed some mutton broth.

Date	Symptoms and Complaints	Comments
	bowel movement (blood?); additional *Mars Hydrarg*, antimony and ipecac. Later that afternoon became febrile, coughing "pinkish mucous."	
March 30	Miller provided more *Mars Hydrarg* as well as ipecac, opium camphor and *Pulvus Rhei*; "voluminous bowel movements; Miller again prescribed additional *Mars Hydrarg*, ipecac camphor and opium.	Spent comfortable night (perhaps due to the opium) and seemed improved by morning; at least the president said he felt better. Later that day became more febrile; pulse 85.
March 31	Miller prescribed *serpentaria* (Virginia snake weed root) and *seneka* (*Polygala senega*) enemas. When Harrison again developed a fever, Miller prescribed periodic doses of *Mars Hydrarg*, ipecac, antimony and spirits of ammonia.	Fewer bowel movements. Cough produced yellowish mucous which contained blood. Fever returned.
April 1	*Mars Hydrarg* applied over surface of abdomen but other medications temporarily discontinued. Frequent bowel movements. Harrison complained of additional pain on right side and above eyebrow. A warm poultice was applied to the side and *Granville's lotion* (counterirritant consisting of rosemary, camphor and ammonia) along the spine, which relieved some of the pain. *Mars Hydrarg*, camphor and opium again administered.	Harrison became incoherent as condition appeared to worsen. Miller requested assistance of additional physicians: Drs. N.W. Worthington of Georgetown and James C. Hall of Washington. The consultants recommended that Miller continue the enemas.
April 2	Harrison began spitting up bloody brownish mucous. Given *blue mass* (mercury) and additional enemas. A "dry hacking cough" was relieved with a dose of	Appeared flushed and febrile. An initially rapid pulse increasingly slowed over the course of the day; extremities became "blue and cold."

Date	Symptoms and Complaints	Comments
	squill (Scilla maratima root), morphia and *Tolu.* At 2:30 p.m. passed "large watery" stool. Given 20 drops of laudanum; abdomen distended. Stimulants and mustard plasters were applied to his extremities, along with starch, laudanum and *kino* (red plant juice) enema, and a hot brandy containing camphor and carbonate of ammonia was provided.	
April 3	Dr. Ashton Alexander of Baltimore added to consultant team. Frequent and feculent discharges exhausted the president, who was given laudanum periodically as well as the mixture of starch, laudanum and *kino.*	Harrison slept periodically and fitfully during the day, occasionally muttering in his sleep. Became languid with difficulty in being aroused. The physicians considered the case increasingly hopeless. At 8:45 p.m. uttered last words: "Sir, I wish you to understand the true principles of government; I wish them carried out, I ask nothing more."
April 4	12:30 a.m.: Harrison died	

Time course of Harrison's illness. Descriptions and quotes based primarily on information provided by McHugh and Mackowiak[26] as well as from the primary source (Miller).[27]

As described in the table, which charts the course of Harrison's illness, the evidence that pneumonia may not have been the initial problem originated three weeks after the inauguration when Harrison, suffering from a fever, "fatigue and anxiety," requested that his doctor, Thomas Miller, come to the White House. Miller already had a history of serving prominent patients, including the family of Martin Van Buren, and would continue in that capacity through the James Buchanan administration. In Miller's words written following the president's death, "the disease was not viewed as a case of pure pneumonia; but as this was the most palpable affection, the term pneumonia afforded a succinct and intelligible answer to the innumerable questions as to the nature of the attack."

The case did not initially seem to be of a critical nature:

On the 26th of March 1841, at 5:00 p.m., I [Dr. Miller] was summoned to visit President Harrison. I found him slightly ailing, although not confined to his room. He complained of having been somewhat indisposed for several days, which he attributed to the great fatigue and mental anxiety he had undergone; stated that he had taken [undisclosed] medicine, had been dieting himself, and believed that he would soon be well again; that he had sent for me, not to prescribe, being his own physician in slight attacks, but to confer with me respecting some of the peculiarities of his constitution, which he thought it important that his physician should be aware of. He mentioned his liability to neuralgia, affecting his head, stomach, and often his extremities; that he had been, early in life, a martyr to dyspepsia; that for the last few years he had avoided these dyspeptic attacks by a system of diet, confining himself principally to animal food; he had been starving himself for a few days past, in consequence of some return of his old dyspepsia; that when sick he always required a very stimulating practice; that he slept but little, going to bed early, and rising very early; that he attributed his good health during the last few years to that circumstance. I advised that he should avoid all excitement, that he should remain quiet the next morning in bed, and intermit his official business, which he promised to do. At his request, I called in the evening at 8 o'clock, found him in his parlor, with several of his old military friends; he informed me that he felt much better than he had done for some days; that he thought he would have a good night, and be well by the morning: he was cheerful, and joined in the conversation.[28]

Several aspects of Miller's description appear relevant here. First, it is apparent that the president had felt ill for several days prior to contacting Dr. Miller. He appeared "somewhat indisposed," a vague description and one which in retrospect could be consistent with the early stages of typhoid (albeit as well as other illnesses). Dyspepsia (difficulty in breathing), from which the president suffered periodically, might also have indicated the early stages of a gastrointestinal illness such as typhoid. Nothing here would indicate an initial diagnosis of cholera (the later description of constipation would appear to rule that out) or pneumonia. Miller treated the president with several of the standard methods of the time: opium and enemas, procedures which could potentially cause perforation of the intestines, allowing pathogens to become systemic. A week later, Harrison was dead.

Could the pneumonia have been a secondary infection? McHugh and Mackowiak present the possibility of an enteric infection based upon several primary sources of evidence. First was the description of the patient himself. As Harrison approached death he exhibited a "sinking pulse" and "cold, blue extremities," characteristics of septic shock. The authors pointed out that while some of the symptoms could be consistent with a diagnosis of pneumonia, fever, dyspnea and sputum tinged with blood, those symptoms did not arise until the fifth day of the illness and even then remained "intermittent." On the other hand, the abdominal discomfort and constipation arose on the third day of the illness. The president's bowels "opened" on the sixth day of his illness, and as McHugh and Mackowiak suggest, this could be the result either of the laxatives or the intestinal damage resulting from the infection. Even the respiratory descriptions were consistent with that of typhoid; again the authors pointed out that such symptoms are often mistaken for symptoms of a respiratory illness.[29]

Perhaps more important in pinpointing the source of the president's infection was the nature of sanitation at the time. As McHugh and Mackowiak point out, the city had no proper sewage system at the time, and it was not unusual for raw sewage to collect in the low-lying marshland. The sewer system in the city, allegedly discharging ground and drain water into local canals or the river, had been largely built by 1810; and though updated periodically, by 1840 it was inadequate for the growing city. In fact, the water supply for the White House was downstream of the depository of "night soil," human feces collected from privies or cesspools. Since typhoid and other enteric fevers were common, it requires minimal imagination to see the water supply utilized by Harrison would likely have been contaminated.

Zachary Taylor (1784–1850)

Zachary Taylor was born November 24, 1784, into a family of Virginia planters and slaveholders. His father, Richard Taylor, had served honorably during the Revolutionary War. The family became relatively wealthy for the times, ultimately owning over 10,000 acres of land in Kentucky near present-day Louisville. Embarking on a career in the military, Zachary received a commission as first lieutenant of a Kentucky regiment in 1808, and by the following year was serving as a temporary commander of Fort Pickering near present-day Memphis. Returning to Louisville in 1810, he married Margaret Mackall Smith, daughter of another wealthy planter.

During the War of 1812, Taylor, now a captain, was in charge of the post at Fort Harrison near present-day Terre Haute, Indiana. It was there that he had his first taste of battle, when the undermanned fort—consisting of approximately sixteen healthy soldiers and others numbering approximately thirty-five laid low by what was likely dysentery or malaria—was attacked in September by several hundred Native Americans. Despite the overwhelming odds and a fire which began when the whiskey supply came under fire, Taylor was able to rally his men and maintain sufficient discipline to beat off the attack. As a result of his calmness in battle, he received a commendation from General William Henry Harrison and a promotion to brevet (temporary) major. Taylor was officially promoted to major as the war came to an end in 1814.

In the ensuing decades Taylor became commander of the fort at Baton Rouge, Louisiana, where he gained renown as an Indian fighter in areas as far west as portions of Texas and as far north as Minnesota and Wisconsin. With the outbreak of the Mexican War in 1846 (indeed, it was President James Knox Polk's order to now General Taylor to enter Mexican territory in present-day southwestern Texas that began the war) Taylor defeated the Mexican army under General Santa Anna, he of Alamo and San Jacinto infamy—in several engagements, including the decisive battle of Buena Vista. By now "Old Rough and Ready," as he became known, was a national hero. In 1848, Taylor and Millard Fillmore headed the Whig Party ticket in the presidential election, defeating Democrat Lewis Cass and free-soiler and former president Martin Van Buren. Taylor himself was a slaveholder and the slavery issue was a major area of contention during Taylor's brief presidency, as it had been for decades. Taylor was largely an advocate of what would become known as popular sovereignty—allowing an incoming state to decide for itself whether to allow slavery—but he was adamant in his belief that secession was illegal. It was Taylor's stance on the slavery issue which was in part the basis for some of the controversy surrounding his death.

Death of Taylor

During the summer of 1850 the most recent epidemic of cholera, one which had begun the year before, was still spreading through the Midwest and East Coast. Though there was little evidence of any significant outbreak in the nation's capital, people were still warned about possible contamination of food or water. On July 4, 1850, a typically hot, humid day in Washington, Taylor participated in the holiday celebrations. He was likely sitting beneath a canopy near the partially completed Washington monument as Senator Henry Foote from Mississippi delivered an address and dust from the tomb of Polish patriot Thaddeus Kosciusko was placed in the monument. Taylor then took a walk along the river for several hours, and upon returning to the White House he consumed a large quantity of cold milk and ice water as well as cherries and other fruit, in retrospect possible sources of infection. Shortly afterwards, he developed severe stomach pains. Despite feeling ill, the following day, July 5, he was well enough to sign a ratification letter for the Clayton-Bulwer Treaty, which established guidelines between the United States and Great Britain over control of a canal across Central America, and to pen a letter to Ezra Prentice, president of the New York State Agricultural Society, about plans to attend the state fair in September. Taylor became increasingly ill with nausea and diarrhea during the following day and was unable to consume food or drink. He had suffered similar symptoms a year earlier, so there was no immediate concern about his condition. However, by the afternoon of July 6, as the family became concerned about Taylor's increasingly severe symptoms, they contacted an army surgeon, Dr. Alexander Wotherspoon, for treatment. The diagnosis was cholera.

The following day, July 7, the first reports and rumors reached the public concerning Taylor's condition. When his body began to reject fluids, including even ice chips, two additional physicians were called in: army surgeon Richard Coolidge and Dr. James Hall. Hall had previously been among the consultants called in during the illness of President Harrison. Taylor became increasingly despondent, telling his doctors, "In two days I shall be a dead man."[30] On the morning of July 9 Taylor told his doctors, "You have fought a good fight, but you cannot make a stand." He later called to his wife, his last words being, "I have always done my duty, I am ready to die. My only regret is for the friends I leave behind me."[31] The diagnosis from the physicians was gastroenteritis, a generic diagnosis which might have referred to any number of illnesses.

The controversy centers on the cause of Taylor's death. Contemporary physicians diagnosed his final illness as cholera morbus—acute cholera. Others believe, as in the focus of this story, that it may have been typhoid fever or at least some form of dysentery. More recently the focus has been on the possibility of arsenic poisoning. Any of these is possible, but a definitive answer is likely impossible with the passage of time. In the following we look at each of these possibilities, beginning with the one which has actually been investigated: arsenic.

The possibility of arsenic poisoning was analyzed during the 1990s, drawing upon modern forensic testing. Impetus for the more complete modern analysis came from Dr. Clara Rising, a retired humanities professor and author from the University of Florida who hoped to find an answer to a question which had long been a rumor, that Taylor had been assassinated by poisoning. Rising agreed to pay the approximately $1,200 cost of exhuming the late president's body and preparing samples for analysis. On June 16, 1991, Jefferson County, Kentucky, coroner Richard Greathouse removed Taylor's (badly deteriorated) coffin from its resting place in Louisville, transporting the remains in a hearse for analysis. The remains were returned to the crypt later in the day.

Samples of hair, bone and fingernail tissue from the body were sent to the Oak Ridge National Laboratory, where two members of the Chemical and Analytical Sciences Division, Larry Robinson and Frank Dyer, using the modern technique of neutron activation analysis, measured the level of arsenic in the samples. Their findings and conclusion, released a week later, were that while trace levels of arsenic were detected—not surprisingly since most persons have such trace levels—no significant quantity of the element was present. There was no evidence that Taylor died from arsenic poisoning.[32]

Others have disputed those findings. According to writer and political activist Michael Parenti, the analysis of Taylor's tissue was incomplete. His argument for arsenic poisoning is largely based on negative evidence: that the symptoms were compatible with such poisoning, as was noted in the original Oak Ridge report, but could also have been the result of other "natural diseases." Fair enough. Parenti also argued that the hair analysis should have been carried out in the "cross-section of hair near the scalp," rather than on the entire piece of hair. Perhaps, but this presupposes the results of the analysis would differ. While possible, arsenic poisoning remains in the area of speculation.[33]

What of the other possibilities for gastroenteritis? The rapid onset of the illness would fit more with a diagnosis of cholera, or even other forms of *Salmonella* infection, rather than typhoid fever. Contemporary accounts indicate the illness began within one day, with no reports of a rash or elevated temperature, certainly not what one might expect if he had suffered from typhoid fever. Finally, in the area of speculation, historian Samuel Eliot Morison has proposed an unintentional "medical assassination." Using the medical arsenal of the time, Wotherspoon may have treated the president with ipecac, calomel (mercury), opium and quinine, in addition to bleeding him. Perhaps this was more than a sixty-six-year-old body could have withstood on top of the actual illness itself.[34] In the end we are forced to abide by the original diagnosis: gastroenteritis. Specific cause is unknown, though symptoms such as the rapid onset of abdominal pain and diarrhea better fit a diagnosis of cholera rather than typhoid.

7

Identifying the Etiological Agent

Before it was even known what typhoid actually was—a poison, gas/miasma, something alive?—the disease became the subject of several public health efforts. The urban crowding that followed on the heels of industrialization triggered epidemics in cities, progressing along contaminated water supplies. Though the worst outbreaks were found in poorer neighborhoods, the rich were not spared. As described in the previous chapter, even Prince Albert likely died from the disease in 1861. While until the 1860s France had led the way in pathology, and made some significant advances in public health beginning in the early decades of the century, concerns about personal freedom overshadowed legislative efforts. In the mind of the most influential French thinker in the field, former surgeon René Louis Villermé, "the poor themselves" brought on disease and the problem was nigh impossible to solve, being rooted in their immoral behavior.[1] But to many British physicians, who had for years been addressing sanitary issues on a local level, for which the centralized French medical establishment did not allow, it was time to act.[2]

Early efforts centered on miasmatic ideas of disease. Edwin Chadwick, appointed by the British Parliament in an attempt to reform the Poor Law system, became convinced as a result of his investigation that vapors produced by rotting material were the root cause of disease and the reason why impoverished persons were often chronically ill. As a result of his lobbying, the Public Health Act was passed in 1848, which allowed the government to require towns with high rates of mortality to create local boards of health.[3] The act met with some opposition, but by the end of the century firmly entrenched legislation allowed for medical officers of health to investigate local outbreaks and empowered them to take action in dealing with unsanitary conditions.

These physicians practiced an epidemiology based more on connections than causes. Conflicting ideas, initially on the source of the contagion but later on its cause, existed without a clear consensus or a means to prove one hypothesis versus another. With the connection between typhoid and filth becoming clear as a result of William Budd's observations of transmission seemingly through feces (Chapter 5), it would seem apparent that this question had been settled even if the agent remained unclear. But Budd's interpretation still underwent a challenge from another prominent British physician, Charles Murchison.

Charles Murchison

By the 1870s Charles Murchison had become an important figure in the study of fevers. Born in Jamaica in 1830 the son of a physician, he was educated in Scotland, to which the family had moved when he was three years old. As with many prominent physicians raised in Scotland, he was educated at the University of Edinburgh, passing the examination to become a surgeon in 1850. After serving several years with the Bengal Army in India and Burma, where he had the opportunity to study disease in that area, he returned to London and practiced there for the remaining years of his life. During the next 20 years Murchison served as physician at several hospitals, including the London Fever Hospital and St. Thomas's Hospital, sites which provided ample opportunities for carrying out his observation and researches on the subject of fevers. Murchison had no argument with the observations of Louis, Gerhard, Budd and others, which demonstrated that typhoid was a unique disease. He acknowledged such in his lengthy work published in 1873: "1. When lenticular rose-spots ... appear in successive crops in the course of continued fever, the abdominal lesions of enteric fever [typhoid] are invariably present. 2. When the eruption of typhus ... shows itself in the course of continued fever, the abdominal lesions of enteric fever are absent."[4] As for the contagious nature of typhoid, Murchison still was not completely convinced:

> Among the greatest benefits that medicine has conferred on the human race is the discovery of the causes of human disease, and of the measures by which they may be prevented. Recent researches have thrown much light on the causes of Continued Fevers, and render it probable that, whether or not these diseases be necessarily in every instance traceable to contagion, their prevalence is to a great extent under human control. The causes vary according to the species of fever, and are equally deserving of study whether they be regarded as predisposing or exciting....
>
> It was contended that we have it in our power, not only to arrest the

spread of continued fevers, but in many cases to prevent their origin. This view has recently been ably advocated by independent observers, such as Virchow, Bence Jones, Beale, Barker, etc.; while, on the contrary, it has excited vigorous opposition on the part of many who seem to argue that if a disease can once be proved to be contagious, it cannot possibly arise in any other way than by contagion, and who maintain that in every instance of the apparently independent origin of such diseases, the introduction of the poison has merely eluded observation, and that the advocates of its independent origin are in the untenable position of attempting to prove a negative. The strongest analogies and figures of speech have been appealed to in denouncing the doctrine of what is called the spontaneous origin of specific diseases. It has been assumed, for example, that contagia are vegetable parasites.... Such premises being taken for granted, it has been argued that the origin *de novo* of a fever poison is as impossible as the spontaneous generation of plants and animals. After mature consideration of the arguments advanced on both sides of this difficult question, the following reasons induce me to adhere to my original [skeptical] opinion:

1. Admitting the parasitic nature of contagious diseases does not exclude the possibility of their independent origin, and for two reasons:—a. [Ernst] Hallier himself states that the two maladies in which he has studied the matter the most, viz. cholera and sheep-pox, may arise independently of pre-existing cases, through the agency of minute fungi growing upon the rice-plant and upon blighted darnel; b. It is still an unsettled question whether certain minute animal and vegetable organisms, such as Bacteria and Vibriones, may not appear *de novo* in organic fluids.

2. The parasitic theory rests solely on analogy and is unsupported by facts.... Contagia no doubt resemble minute organisms in being endowed with the power of rapid self-multiplication and in retaining their vitality out of the body, but the highest powers of the microscope have hitherto failed to show that the spread of any of the acute specific diseases is due to the presence of such organisms. It is true that Bacteria and Vibriones—*microzymes* as they have been called—have been found in the blood of enteric fever, malignant pustule, and allied diseases; but it is equally true that they are absent from many fluids possessing virulent contagious properties, and common enough in fluids which are known to be harmless. Their presence is therefore probably the consequence, rather than the cause, of disease.

3. Although the mode of introduction of a contagium often eludes observation, yet if all contagious diseases can arise in no other way than by contagia, their germs must be both omnipresent and indestructible by time; and it is difficult to conceive how so many persons escape them. Their not furnishing a suitable soil does not suffice to account for their immunity. Moreover, on this supposition, the germs of certain diseases, such as enteric fever, would require to be much more potent than they have yet been shown to be, to account for the circumstances under which these diseases often appear.[5]

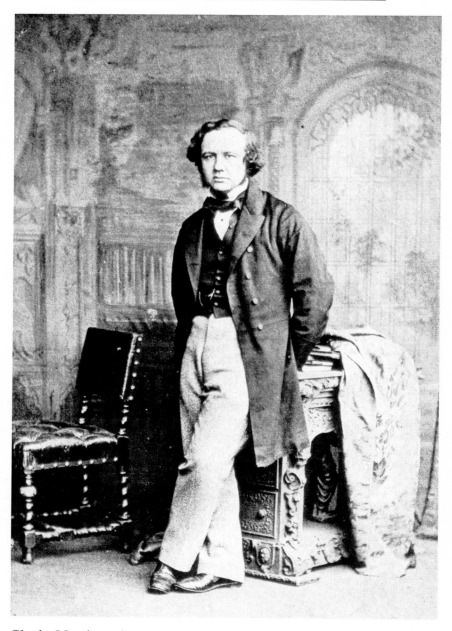

Charles Murchison (1830–1879), British physician noted for his study of fevers. His work, *A Treatise on the Continued Fevers of Great Britain* (1862), was considered at the time as the authoritative work on the subject (courtesy Wellcome Library, London).

Murchison continued with other reasons he was not yet firmly convinced of what, within a few years, would be the "germ theory of disease." Ignorant of the existence of viruses and living in a time where the theory of evolution and the nascent field of bacteriology were still in their infancy, it is understandable that Murchison was unable to completely discount the idea that microorganisms, or at least the diseases they caused, might appear spontaneously. To him, typhoid could certainly be transmitted between people, but seemingly novel (*de novo*) appearances of the disease could not be explained through that fact alone. He believed that the disease-causing agent could be produced much like a chemical byproduct, "the degraded offspring" of feces that was breaking down.[6]

Sometimes the source of typhoid was more indirect than that of contaminated drinking water. In these cases, investigators had to think creatively, looking to other possible vehicles of transmission. Ironically, Murchison himself had an opportunity to observe such a connection between contaminated liquids and an epidemic of typhoid. An outbreak in 1873 involved a district in London with clean water and decent drainage: Marylbone, where Murchison, William Jenner and a number of other physicians lived.[7] Five of Murchison's children became ill and, knowing that the water supply was not to blame, he pointed towards the local supplier of milk, the Dairy Reform Company. There was precedent for his suspicions. In 1870 a medical health officer, Edward Ballard, had published a pamphlet about outbreaks of typhoid associated with milk. Ballard had investigated a previous outbreak and noted how it had been limited to the wealthy rather than the poor. The disease appeared only in households which obtained their milk from a particular dairy, and only in those members who drank the milk. Individuals and even whole families living under the same roof were spared if they had not drunk the milk. Milk, Ballard reasoned, could be contaminated through being watered down or through being handled in pails that had been washed with dirty water.[8]

The Dairy Reform Company insisted that their milk was not watered down, and investigation by a local health officer suggested that the blame lay at one or more of their supplier farms. A six-person group, including health officer John Radcliffe, two company representatives and other authorities visited each of eight supplier farms. Seven had adequate sanitation, while the eighth was revealed to have had several individuals with cases of typhoid. The disease had even claimed the owner of the farm, and upon advice from a physician, well-meaning family members had made sure to deposit his feces in an ash heap away from the privy, concerned that their vapors might spread the disease. This was found to be "perhaps the only spot on the farm premises where they would certainly find their way into the water used for dairy purposes," because a leaking drain allowed for material from the ash heap and nearby pigsty to mix with the well water. The Dairy Reform Company was forced to acknowledge that their milk had been contaminated and instated regular inspections of its farms.[9]

Despite the life-threatening illnesses, Murchison believed the "Marylbone milk crisis," as it was called by the British press, still produced benefits for the public: first, that typhoid was not only waterborne, but that milk might also serve as a vehicle; second, that as a result of the outbreak, legislation to curb unsanitary dairy practices was passed; and third, that consumers became aware of the danger of "adulterated milk."[10]

The Germ Theory of Disease: The French Contribution

The modern understanding of the germ theory of disease—the concept that (infectious) disease is the result of the presence of microscopic organisms within the organism regardless of how they were acquired—had its origins in the mid to latter nineteenth century. While the French chemist Louis Pasteur and German physician Robert Koch are acknowledged to have been the key players in development of the theory, this is not to say that similar ideas had not appeared much earlier. But there is a significant difference between the hypothesis produced by an observer, regardless of how accurate it may have been proven at a later time, and the technology necessary to prove the postulate. The development and evolution of the microscope is a prime model. For example, the Italian Girolamo Fracastoro, the sixteenth century Italian physician and scholar, proposed as early as the 1540s that tiny entities might be the cause of disease and that contagion was the result of their transfer between humans. His hypothesis, while substantially correct, could not be proven. While the Dutch tradesman and lensmaker Antonie van Leeuwenhoek developed one of the early functional microscopes a century later, even observing microscopic organisms, which likely included larger bacteria, the work was never connected with disease.

During the early to mid-nineteenth century numerous examples of what in retrospect could have evolved into the germ theory were studied, the observations of Bretonneau, Louis, Gerhard and others discussed earlier. Perhaps the most notable was the work of the English physician John Snow in his study of cholera outbreaks in London in 1849 and 1854. While he did not isolate and identify the etiological agent, he did demonstrate in each instance a link between sewage contaminated water and the epidemics.

And there was the key, the inability to demonstrate the role of a microscopic agent and the disease.

Louis Pasteur never experimented directly with typhoid fever despite the fact three of his children died from that malady. But his work set the foundation for the germ theory. A chemist by training—and perhaps it should be kept in mind that Pasteur's work fell in that scientific category—he began his career studying crystalline structures, discovering that some molecules were structurally mirror images of each other. He noted the same property in molecules from living organisms.[11]

During the 1860s, many prominent physicians and scientists still believed microorganisms could arise in decaying matter. For some, like Murchison, who clearly perceived that typhoid, cholera and other waterborne diseases were associated with fecal contamination, this idea of de novo creation of microscopic organisms made both theoretical and practical sense: gaps in the chain of transmission could be explained; and purifying the waste using disinfectants, presumably destroying whatever

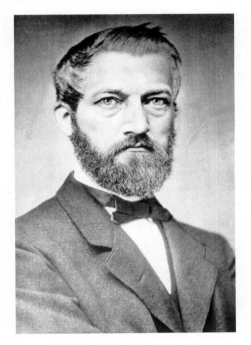

Louis Pasteur (1822–1895), French chemist and bacteriologist who, along with the German Robert Koch, was a key figure in development of the Germ Theory of Disease. A brief listing of Pasteur's accomplishments would include development of the first vaccines against anthrax and rabies and the refutation of spontaneous generation (courtesy National Library of Medicine).

life force was present, prevented additional cases from occurring. In France, this same idea was broadly proposed by Felix-Archimède Pouchet, a strong proponent of spontaneous generation. Pouchet believed that new life appeared in waste as the result of a strange "plastic force" which enabled organic molecules to spontaneously assemble into life forms.[12]

Pouchet's approach to spontaneous generation was not well received as the concept came to sound not only unscientific but suspiciously sacrilegious—removing a creator god from the story of life and replacing him with a less purposeful force.[13] Regardless of the growing scientific opposition, Pouchet published his hypotheses in a book, *Heterogenie* (1859), which drew added attention towards his views. In turn, the French academy of sciences offered a monetary prize to anyone who could refute Pouchet or "throw new light" on the issue.[14]

Pasteur was not strongly religious, but he was driven by a desire for acclaim and dedication to his science. He already had objections to the idea of spontaneous generation prior to the Académie's offer: the idea seemed dangerously subversive to his conservative sensibilities and, the result of his previous work—his determination that microorganisms were the cause of fermentation reactions, not their product. Pasteur conducted a series of experiments to demonstrate that organisms were not produced by decaying matter but that they were introduced from the air. His experimental design was relatively simple. Swan-necked flasks which contained nutrient-enriched water which had been boiled were sealed. In the absence of outside air, no growth occurred. If the necks were broken and air was introduced, growth took place. In his public lecture during which he described his results, Pasteur reported that "I have removed from [the nutrient mixture] the only thing that it has not been given man to produce.... I have removed life, for life is the germ, and the germ is life."[15]

Proving, at least in minds of most persons, that microorganisms were ubiquitous and that air was a common source of contamination was one thing. Proving that these same microorganisms might be the agents of disease was a greater challenge. As recounted earlier, by the late 1860s physicians were already making a connection between microbes and illness. Since the atmosphere already contained "invisible" organisms, the idea could quickly merge with the concept of miasmas or "emanations," the result of putrefaction, as the agents of those diseases. Microorganisms themselves were the agents of putrefaction.

Among the first to apply in a medical practice the concept of environmental microbes as the etiological agents of disease was British surgeon Sir Joseph Lister. After becoming aware of Pasteur's experiments, Lister began the practice of not only disinfecting his medical instruments with carbolic acid, but also treating the dressings of surgical wounds with a similar solution. During surgery, Lister arranged for an assistant to spray the solution in the area of the operation, further reducing the danger of infection. By 1875 a new term was coined defining Lister's technique: antisepsis.

Louis Pasteur (1822–1895)

Louis Pasteur was born in Dole, France, in 1822, the third child (of five) of Jean-Joseph Pasteur, a tanner and decorated veteran of Napoleon's army. After his primary education at Collegé d'Arbois, where his family had moved when he was five, Pasteur entered the Institution Barbet in Paris (1838), a preparatory school which would ideally lead to admission at the prestigious École Normale Supérieure. Homesick, however, he returned home within several months. The following year he enrolled in Collége Royal de Basençon in eastern France, completing a course in philosophy needed for admission to the normal school. In 1840 he graduated with a bachelor of arts degree, remaining at the school for further training in science as well as teaching mathematics and serving as a tutor. In 1844 he was enrolled at École Normale Supérieure, graduating with a bachelor of science the following year. Pasteur continued to pursue studies in chemistry at the École Normale, earning his doctorate in 1847 with theses in both chemistry and physics.[16]

After brief service in the national guard during the 1848 revolution in Paris and a brief sojourn at the lycée in Dijon, Pasteur was appointed professor of chemistry at the University of Strasbourg, subsequently being appointed to the chair of chemistry. In addition to his initial research on the subject of optical activity which he carried out, Pasteur's personal life was enhanced with his marriage to Marie Laurent, daughter of the rector of the Strasborg Academy. They would have five children, three of whom died from typhoid fever.

In 1857 Pasteur moved to Paris, where he was appointed director of scientific studies at the École Normale Supérieure, site of his earlier studies. It was here where he began the research which would establish his role as one of the founders of germ theory. His early work involved the study of fermentation, which he demonstrated could be carried out by a particular microorganism—yeast. Within a few years he demonstrated the role of different microorganisms in fermentation and spoilage of milk, beer and wine, eventually proposing a possible role for such organisms in the human body. But a series of student revolts on the issue of free thought, combined with Pasteur's dissatisfaction with the political bent of the school, resulted in its temporary closing and his own firing. But by this time Pasteur's prestige was such that he was too valuable to simply be replaced. The Ministry of Public Instruction offered him a professorship in chemistry at the Sorbonne, and under pressure from the emperor, Louis Napoleon, a laboratory for the study of physiological chemistry was to be built at the École Normale, with Pasteur allowed to carry out research as he wished.[17] He would remain director for twenty years, before moving to the newly established Pasteur Institute in 1888.

Pasteur's research on the subject of infectious disease is well known and has been the subject of several excellent texts.[18] A very brief overview illustrates the depth of his work, the success of which was the result of his "workaholic" nature. Nothing in his laboratory was carried out without his direct oversight. Pasteur's initial research in this area resulted in a vaccine against chicken cholera in 1880. During the late 1870s he also began working on a vaccine for protecting animals against anthrax, a significant problem in the largely rural economy. Using what we now understand as a heat inactivation technique, he was able to produce an analogous vaccine against that latter disease. In a famous field trial held during the early summer 1881 at Pouilly-le-Fort, Pasteur demonstrated the efficacy of the vaccine in protecting sheep exposed to the anthrax bacillus. In an address before the Academy of Sciences that June, Pasteur linked the two successes: "In sum, we now possess some virus-vaccines of anthrax, capable of providing protection against the fatal disease without ever being fatal themselves, living vaccines, cultivatable at will, transportable anywhere without alteration, and, lastly, prepared by a method that one may consider capable of generalization since it served a previous time for the discovery of the chicken cholera vaccine. By virtue of the conditions I have enumerated here, and to look at things solely from the scientific point of view, the discovery of these anthrax vaccines constitutes a considerable advance over the Jennerian vaccine against smallpox, for the latter has never been obtained experimentally."[19] In this last sentence Pasteur pointed out that, while the vaccine produced by Edward Jenner was a naturally attenuated form of a similar virus, both the chicken cholera and anthrax vaccines were created in the laboratory, the first such to have been produced in that manner.

Pasteur's most famous success was his development of a vaccine against rabies, a disease transmitted through the saliva of a rabid animal. While not a particularly common disease, the fact that the victim would suffer horribly from the invariably fatal infection made it one of the most feared illnesses. Pasteur's research during 1884 and 1885 resulted in production of a vaccine using dried spinal cord tissue from experimentally infected animals. His successful treatment in July 1885 of a boy, Joseph Meister, who had been badly mauled by a rabid dog, became known throughout the world.

Soon after the successful trials with the rabies vaccines, age and cardiovascular problems forced Pasteur to retire from research. The Pasteur Institute was completed in 1888, but by then Pasteur was too ill to participate in more than its dedication. He died in 1895.

One of the phenomena of typhoid fever, indeed of any of the contagious diseases, which researchers had to explain was that of the incubation period. Because they were conditioned to think of disease as being the result of poisons of some sort, physicians often presumed that symptoms should appear shortly after the bacteria entered the body. Budd had proposed one possible reason for the delay:

> Taking cognizance of the fact that physicians, nurses and other attendants upon the sick are often remarkably exempt from infection, and that, consequently, the contagious matter as it appears in the dejections upon their issue from the body, is not probably in a condition favorable to the manifestation of immediate activity,—he [Budd] held that it requires to undergo some changes, outside the body, to fit it for transmission. It was his idea that when first cast of it is, so to speak, in bulk; that it appears in the discharges in the form of "clots or pellets of yellow matter" which are "to the contagious germs that float impalpable in air or water much as the block of granite is to the dust into which it may be ground," and that before it can exert to its full extent the contagious power inherent in it, the infective germ or particle must be liberated from its entanglements and the organic husks in which it is embedded, by drying, fermentation, or some other mode of disintegration or subdivision.[20]

Budd's hypothesis of "clots or pellets" undergoing disintegration at least explained the efficacy of disinfection. Carl von Liebermeister, German pathologist noted for his study of fevers, envisioned some form of life cycle for the organism in explaining the incubation period. Liebermeister "maintained that it [the typhoid organism] multiplies in the body and is contained in the alvine [intestinal] evacuations.... It requires for the full development of its infective powers to undergo a stage of growth and multiplication outside the body, in connection with decomposing animal and vegetable matter, such as eminently it finds in privies, and cesspools, and sewers.... The poison travels from the diseased individual to localities favorable to its growth and multiplication, and from these localities again into the human body."[21] In the viewpoint of Liebermeister, the time necessary for growth in the victim wasn't the issue but the time that the organism spent in the medium whose stench or chemistry had long been indicated as potential sources.

Clarity on this subject could only result from studying the microorganism itself. For researchers to do that, they had to first isolate the microbe and link it to the specific disease. During the first years in which Pasteur began his work, the ability to carry this out was hampered by technological limitations. Most bacteria could be grown easily enough using nutrient broths or on food items such as bread, starchy vegetables (potato) or meat. But it was still difficult to separate the colonies of different species. Even observing bacteria was a challenge, as the lens system of the period was still limited in its resolving power. Final proof for the germ theory of disease would result from a shift from French research to the nascent German school of work in that area.

The Germ Theory of Disease: The German Contribution

During the first half of the century a large proportion of the medical investigation in Europe had taken place in France. This was about to change, as, beginning in the 1870s, Germany began to surpass France in the level and quality of bacteriological research. The reasons varied but included factors such as an increase in support for such work and significant improvement and freedom in universities where much of the work would be carried out. Scientific competition among the professors was encouraged, and the schools established high standards in regard to testing and admission requirements. The unification of the country under Otto von Bismarck in 1871 played no small role in the process.

The changing scientific climate was a boon to Robert Koch, who had begun his medical career as a country doctor and *Kreisphysikus*, a health officer, the latter in hopes of earning a decent living in his profession. Koch's interest in bacteriological research began partly by chance. In 1873 an outbreak of anthrax in the district of Bomst, then in eastern Germany but now within Poland, allowed Koch to microscopically examine samples of blood from dead cattle.[22] The presence of bacteria in the blood of animals sick with the disease had long been known by then. In 1850 French physician Casimir Davaine and his colleague, the pathologist Pierre Rayer, reported the presence of rod-shaped bacteria in the blood of sheep infected with anthrax, while others described similar organisms in cattle with the disease. Davaine later demonstrated the transmissibility of the organisms: blood taken from a sick animal and injected into a healthy one would induce anthrax in the latter. While in retrospect these experiments provided support for the germ theory, the inability to link these *specific* organisms with this *specific* disease left it to others to develop this theory. Koch described more than simply the presence of bacteria in his samples (April 1874). "The bacteria swell up, become shinier, thicker, and much longer. Slight bends develop. Gradually a thick felt develops. Within the long cells, cross walls appear and small transparent points develop at regular intervals."[23] Koch had observed the formation of endospores, a dormant form of the organism which accounted for their ability to survive extreme environmental conditions.

In December 1875 Koch found further opportunities to study the organism soon known as *Bacillus anthracis,* and in doing so produced a significant advance in the study of disease. Examining a sample of blood from the hide of an animal which had died from anthrax, Koch observed the presence of large numbers of bacteria. A small quantity of the blood was inoculated into a rabbit, which within a day was also dead from anthrax. Microscopic examination of fluid taken from lymph glands in the dead rabbit again revealed the presence of bacteria. Koch again transferred the infectious material, this time into the corneal fluid in the eye of another rabbit. Again the rabbit died, and Koch found bacteria to be present throughout the dead animal. But the same experiment suggested to Koch that the corneal fluid of the eye might also serve as a medium to grow pure cultures of bacteria.[24]

The use of the aqueous humor of the eye represented the first means for the study of isolated microorganisms. There were obvious disadvantages to the procedure (not least of which for the laboratory animal). In the early 1880s Koch improved on this technique by growing bacteria in a nutrient broth to which gelatin was added as a hardening agent. This eliminated the need for using an animal but had the disadvantage of liquefying when incubated at body temperature.[25] Further refinement of Koch's culture method involved replacing the gelatin with another hardening agent, agar, an extract from a type of algae, which would remain a gel at that temperature. What still remained for Koch was to demonstrate the life cycle of the bacterium and confirm its role as the etiological agent of anthrax—key components of what would be the germ theory:

> We thus see that anthrax tissues, regardless of whether they are relatively fresh, putrefying, or years old, can produce anthrax when these substances contain bacilli capable of developing spores of *Bacillus anthracis.* Thus, all doubts regarding *Bacillus anthracis* as the actual cause of the disease must be expelled. *Bacillus anthracis* is indeed the contagion of anthrax. The transmission of the disease in fresh blood occurs rarely in nature, only in persons who come in contact with blood or tissue juices while killing, cutting, and skinning animals infected with anthrax.... But, the great percentage of infections are produced only by the penetration of the spores of *Bacillus anthracis* into the animal body. For the spores can survive in an amazing manner for many years. When these spores have once formed in the soil of a region, there is good reason to believe that anthrax will remain in this region for many years.[26]

Koch's hypothesis was presented to Ferdinand Cohn, a biologist at the University of Breslau and an authority on spores as a part of the life cycle of bacilli. Cohn confirmed Koch's ideas, and with their publication in 1876, Koch achieved his first measure of national fame.[27]

During the 1880s Koch achieved international fame for his isolation and identification of the etiological agents of tuberculosis, for which he was awarded a Nobel Prize in 1905, and cholera. But, arguably, his most famous and lasting contribution lay in developing the procedures sometimes used in linking an etiological agent with a disease: Koch's Postulates. The concept of the postulates actually preceded Koch, originating with the ideas of German pathologist Edwin Klebs: "1. Careful microscopic study of the diseased organ; 2. Isolation and culture of the germ associated with the disease; 3. Production of the same disease by inoculation of this cultured germ into healthy animals."[28] Once Koch developed a method to grow bacteria in pure culture, a component of the postulates which eluded Klebs, the postulates could evolve into the form with which we are familiar today. Ironically it was not Koch himself who published the phraseology initially, but his associate Friedrich Loeffler, in reference to the identification of the diphtheria bacillus: "If diphtheria is a disease caused by a microorganism, it is essential that three postulates be fulfilled. The fulfillment of these postulates is necessary in order to demonstrate strictly the parasitic nature of a disease: 1. The organism must be shown to be constantly present in characteristic form and arrangement in the disease; 2. The organism which, from its behavior appears to be responsible for the disease, must be isolated and grown in pure culture; 3. The pure culture must be shown to induce the disease experimentally." The publication by Koch himself of the postulates occurred later.[29]

Robert Koch (1843–1910)

If one had to choose the single most important figure in development of the germ theory of disease, that choice would likely be Robert Koch. Koch was born in 1843 in Clausthal, the third of 13 children. His father, Hermann Koch, was a successful mining engineer who eventually headed the mining company. As a youth, Koch demonstrated an interest in subjects such as biology and photography. After graduation from the local gymnasium (school), Koch enrolled at the University of Göttingen, from which he received a medical degree in 1866. Among the professors with whom he had the opportunity to interact was Jacob Henle, German physician and anatomist who was an early advocate of what became the germ theory. While attending the university, Koch received a monetary award for a study he carried out under the direction of another professor, Wilhelm Krause, director of the Pathological-Anatomical Institute, entitled "Ueber das Vorkommen von Ganglienzellen an den Nerven des Uterus" (On the Presence of Ganglion Cells on the Nerves of the Uterus), and dedicated the work to his father.[30] Koch continued his taste for research with a study of succinic acid development and excretion in the body in a work titled "Ueber das Entstehen der Bernsteinsäure im menschlichen Organismus." The report was published in 1865 and served as the thesis for his doctoral dissertation.[31]

Koch used the award money he received to travel to Berlin in order to attend the meeting of the Gesellschaft Deutscher Naturforscher und Arzte (Society of Naturalists and Doctors) and carry out further chemical studies. Among those present who would have an influence on his future work was Rudolf Virchow, the physician considered the father of modern pathology and for decades a major figure in scientific research in many areas. Returning home after several months, Koch became engaged to and married Emmy Fraatz, daughter of an official in the church at Clausthal. They would have one daughter, Gertrud, in a marriage which became increasingly unhappy as time passed.[32] During the Franco-Prussian War, which began in 1870, Koch served as a physician in a field hospital, gaining experience in his profession and observing typhoid fever while at a hospital in Neufchâteau. But needed back in the town, Rakwitz, where he had settled with his family before the war, he left the army to resume his practice.[33]

A summary of some of Koch's accomplishments is provided above. In addition to his study of anthrax, Koch was the key figure in isolation and identification of several etiological agents: tuberculosis (1882) and cholera (1884). This does not even include those agents isolated by his associates or students. In 1885, Koch was appointed Professor of Hygiene at the University of Berlin, a position which served as a destination for numerous budding physicians and researchers from many countries during the next decade. In 1900 the Robert Koch (Royal Prussian) Institute for Infectious Diseases was established, an institution which continues today as a site of medical research. Even with his successes, Koch's personal life was in shambles. In 1893 he was divorced, soon after which he married an aspiring actress named Hedwig Freiberg, a woman thirty years younger than he.

Koch was the recipient of numerous awards, most notably the Nobel Prize in Physiology or Medicine in 1905 for his work with tuberculosis. He died from a heart attack in 1910.

Identification of the Etiological Agent of Typhoid Fever

The significance of typhoid fever as a public health problem meant there was no shortage of investigators attempting to determine the cause.

With the development of the germ theory of disease by the 1870s and 1880s the consensus among most physicians was that the agent was a bacterium. As with many scientific discoveries, the issue of priority for its identification is in a gray area.

Perhaps the first to actually report the presence of the typhoid agent was the Polish scientist Tadeusz Browicz, professor of pathologic anatomy at Jagellonian University. In 1874 Browicz described short, rod-shaped organisms he observed in the organs of typhoid victims, as well as in their feces. He was able to isolate and grow the bacteria, indicating their viability. But in these early years of development of the germ theory, Borowicz never attempted to ascertain the pathogenic potential of his isolates.[34]

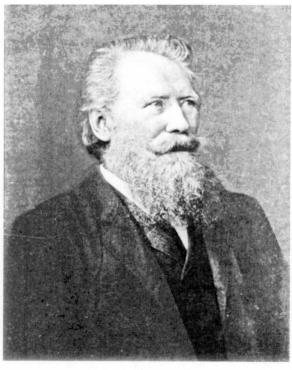

Credit for actual identification of the typhoid bacillus has historically been given to the German pathologist Karl Eberth, who in 1880 observed short, rod-shaped bacteria in the Peyer's patches, mesenteric lymph nodes and other sites in 18 of 40 postmortem examinations of typhoid victims. None of bacteria were observed in "controls" dying from other causes. Eberth also described other organisms as being present, including filamentous bacteria.[35] On occasion, Eberth also reported the presence of what appeared to him as spores. Whether these were truly spores or artifacts of the staining procedure is unknown.[36]

The question of priority might also have been credited to the aforemen-

Karl Eberth (1835–1926). Though it remains questionable whether Eberth was actually the first to observe and describe the etiological agent of typhoid fever, *Eberthella* became the initial name for that bacillus. Photograph taken when he was a young man (courtesy National Library of Medicine).

tioned Edwin Klebs. In April 1880, three months prior to Eberth's claim, Klebs observed both short bacilli as well as filamentous forms in the Peyer's patches of typhoid victims. But as with Browicz before him, their role in the disease was never determined.[37]

In 1881 Koch published the first photomicrographs of bacteria, pictures which included the organisms observed by both Klebs and Eberth. Both agreed the images produced by Koch were identical to those they had seen in the Peyer's patches. Klebs' report has been criticized for describing filamentous forms even though his emphasis was on the short bacilli and that under certain conditions the typhoid agent has been shown to form filaments.[38]

In 1884 the German physician Georg Gaffky, an associate of Koch's, as with most of the key figures in the study of typhoid in the 1880s, isolated the organism from the spleen of a typhoid patient and grew it on solid media.[39] Gaffky was never able to fulfill the third of what we now refer to as Koch's postulates, the induction of the disease in a healthy animal following exposure to the agent. But the fact that it could be found in nearly all cases of typhoid provided strong support for its role as the etiological agent. In recognition of Eberth's (credited) observance in 1880, the organism was given the genus name *Eberthella*.

8

Widal versus Grünbaum: A Question of Priority

> If the reaction takes place rapidly, the first glance through the microscope reveals the completed reaction, all the bacilli being in loose clumps and nearly or altogether motionless. Between the clumps are clear spaces containing few or no isolated bacilli.
>
> If the reaction is a little less complete, a few bacilli may be found moving slowly between the clumps, in an aimless way, while others attached to the clumps by one end are apparently trying to pull away, much as a fly caught on fly-paper struggles for freedom.[1]

The question of priority in discoveries or development of new techniques has always been an issue in the sciences, no less so in the specific area of biology. As we have already seen, while the association of a specific etiological agent with typhoid fever is generally credited to Karl Eberth, one could also make a similar argument on the issue of priority in favor of Edwin Klebs or even the Polish scientist Tadeusz Browicz. Neither, of course, demonstrated the pathogenic ability associated with the organisms they had observed.

The significance of what was known as humoral immunity, the ability of soluble substances in serum to agglutinate or inactivate microbial agents, was among the more prominent areas of scientific conflict between the French and German research communities during the latter years of the nineteenth century.[2] Members of the French medical community were proponents of what became known as cellular immunity. Largely from the work of the Russian born biologist Elie Metchnikoff, by then working at the Pasteur Institute in Paris, "cellularists" argued the major component of the body's immune system was the population of white cells known as macrophages and microphages (neutrophils). The German school, led by

Robert Koch and his associates in Berlin, known as "humoralists," supported the theory that the above-mentioned soluble substances in the blood served as the major components of immunity.

A more detailed discussion of the political background to the competition than is necessary here, as well as experimental data in support of their respective theories, is included in the review by Silverstein.[3] Still, it is helpful to provide the background to the subsequent work carried out by Widal and Grünbaum in developing a diagnostic test for typhoid fever. In 1888 George Nuttall reported that the serum from unimmunized animals possessed bactericidal activity.[4] The bactericidal substance was subsequently termed alexin, later to be termed as complement, by Koch's associate at the Berlin Institute, Paul Ehrlich. Another of Koch's and Ehrlich's associates, Richard Pfeiffer (1858–1945), while working with the cholera agent, observed that fluids from immunized animals had a significantly greater bactericidal effect, a process known as the Pfeiffer phenomenon, in which the organisms undergo swelling, and subsequent lysis.[5] The bactericidal ability could even be passed from an immunized animal to a normal animal using the serum.[6] Behring and another associate of Koch, the Japanese bacteriologist Kitasato Shibasaburo, were able to demonstrate that immunity against diseases such as diphtheria and tetanus would also result from the transfer of serum from an immunized animal. The soluble substances in the serum would become known as antibodies (anti-körper). The bactericidal effects of immune serum, including its effect on typhoid infection, would become well known by the 1890s:

> As a result of investigations covering a period of a year and a half, conducted in conjunction with [Herbert Edward] Durham of London, [Max von] Gruber of Vienna has found that a high degree of long-continuing immunity may be conferred upon guinea-pigs by the intraperitoneal injection of cultures of cholera bacilli, of typhoid bacilli, and of the bacilli coli communes rendered innocuous by chloroform, or by being heated to 140°. The immunity thus conferred relates to infection and not intoxication. The destruction of the bacteria in actively immunized animals, as well as those protected by means of the serum of immune animals, is attributable to the activity of the bodily fluids, the polynuclear phagocytes [i.e., Metchnikoff's theory] playing only a secondary role. The blood and fluids of immune animals contain anti-bodies, which act within the bodies of actively and passively immune persons in the same way as they act outside. In a passively immune person no reactive transformation of the anti-bodies takes place. These anti-bodies have nothing directly to do with the destruction of the bacteria, which takes place as a result of the action of the alexins always present in the bodily fluids. The essential action of the anti-bodies consists in causing the bodies of the bacteria to undergo swelling, as manifested by

stickiness. For this reason the anti-bodies may be designated glabrificins. As a result of the swelling of the bacteria the alexins can gain entrance to their bodies, and thus cause their destruction.[7]

By the 1890s the presence of soluble substances, still referred to as antibodies (the term glabrificins may represent an interesting designation to the medical historian, but it no longer appears in the literature), was clearly recognized as well as the ability of those substances to attach to and neutralize bacteria.

Max von Gruber (1853–1927) and Herbert Edward Durham (1866–1945)

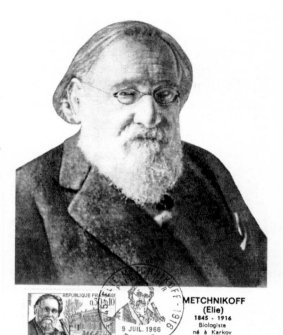

Elie Metchnikoff (1845–1916), Russian born bacteriologist and a key figure in understanding the role of phagocytic cells in the immune response. Much of his professional life was spent at the Pasteur Institute in Paris (courtesy National Library of Medicine).

Born in Vienna, Max von Gruber was a member of a distinguished family of medical practitioners. His father, Ignaz Gruber, was a physician with a specialty in otology, problems associated with the ear (in 1838 he had developed the first tunnel-shaped ear specula composed of a metal). The elder Gruber also authored and published a two-volume text on the subject of medicinal chemistry [*Grundzuge der Allgemeinen und Medicinischen Chemie: ... Band, Welcher die Allgemeine und die Specielle Chemie der Unorganischen Korper Enthalt* (Basic Features of General Medicinal Chemistry...), 1835]. Max Gruber's older brother, Franz von Gruber, joined the military, where he subsequently became a professor at the Imperial and Royal Military Technical Academy. Although Franz was not a trained physician, his work, both in the military and in later life, included the design of hospital buildings, in part influenced by his brother's expertise in hygiene.

Max von Gruber received his medical degree in 1876 from the University of Vienna, following which he studied under the supervision of chemist and hygienist Max von Pettenkofer. In 1884, Gruber was appointed as chairman of the Institute of Hygiene at the University of Graz. Returning to Vienna in 1887, he was subsequently appointed to the chair of the Institute of Hygiene at the University of Vienna. Among Gruber's students in Vienna was the English bacteriologist Herbert Durham (1866–1925) who had been honored with a Sir William Gull studentship. Their collaboration became the basis for the Gruber-Durham agglutination reactions applied first by Richard Pfeiffer and Wilhelm Kolle and subsequently by Fernand Widal and Albert Grünbaum in the identification of typhoid bacilli (see below). It was likely Gruber who first introduced the term agglutinin in identifying the substances in the blood responsible for the reaction. In 1902 Gruber left Vienna for the position of director of the Institute of Hygiene in Munich, where he spent the remainder of his professional career.

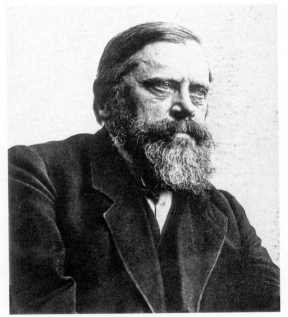

Herbert Durham is remembered for his development of the Durham tube in 1897—used by students of microbiology for generations to detect gas production by bacteria—rather than for his significant contribution to early applications of an agglutination test for identification of bacteria.[8] His father, Dr. Arthur Edward Durham, was senior surgeon at Guy's Hospital in London. Among the elder Durham's accomplishments was the establishment of the Durham prize, awarded to first- and second-year students for expertise in dissection.

Herbert Durham

Max von Gruber (1853–1927). An Austrian bacteriologist, Gruber and his colleague, Herbert Durham, observed the ability of immune serum to agglutinate specific types of bacteria. The procedure was adapted both as a diagnostic tool, and as a means to identify bacteria (courtesy Wellcome Library, London).

attended University College School, followed by King's College in Cambridge, where he qualified for first-class honors in the natural sciences. After working for two years as assistant demonstrator in histology in the physiological laboratory at Cambridge, he joined the staff at Guy's Hospital for clinical work. In 1894 he received a fellowship at the Royal College of Surgeons (FRCS), which qualified him for a position as surgeon. While at Guy's Hospital Durham was awarded the Gull scholarship, allowing him to travel to Vienna, where he carried out his work with Gruber. The results of the Gruber-Durham test (the name went through several alterations before first the Gruber-Widal test and then simply Widal became the standard nomenclature) were presented to the British Royal Society by Durham's mentor and colleague in London, future Nobel laureate Sir Charles

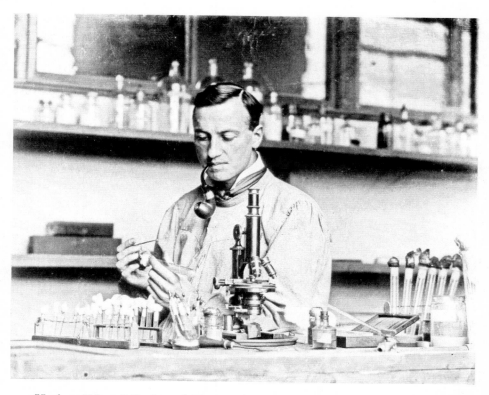

Herbert Edward Durham (1866–1945), British physician who, while working with Max von Gruber, was among the first to observe the agglutinating ability of immune serum. The procedure was adapted by Widal in its use as a diagnostic tool. The Durham tube, which he helped develop, was later used to detect gas production by bacteria (courtesy Wellcome Library, London).

Sherrington. Following his preliminary work on the use of the agglutination procedure as a diagnostic tool, Durham returned to Liverpool and left the remainder of the work to Gruber. As we shall see below, this area of research would be superseded by that of Grünbaum and Widal. Durham's subsequent professional work involved the study of disease carried by the tsetse fly and a subsequent investigation of yellow fever in South America.

It would shortly become evident that the test could be applied for diagnostic purposes. In the studies carried out by Gruber and his student Durham several years earlier (ca. 1894), it was observed that cholera bacilli would undergo agglutination when mixed with fluids obtained from a guinea pig which had been infected with that disease.[9] However, it was Pfeiffer who first proposed that substances in the serum of animals (including humans) exposed to the bacteria not only might provide a measure of immunity but might also be used to demonstrate actual exposure to that organism:

> [Pfeiffer] described a peculiar phenomenon when a portion of a fresh culture of the cholera-vibrion on agar is added to a small quantity of the serum of an animal immunized against cholera, and the mixture injected into the peritoneal cavity of a non-immunized guinea-pig. After this procedure, if

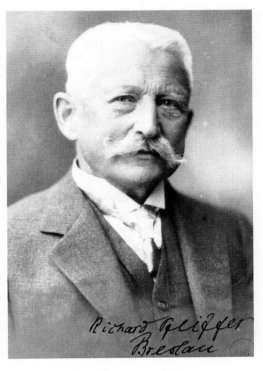

Richard Friedrich Pfeiffer (1858–1945), German physician and bacteriologist and colleague of Robert Koch. Pfeiffer was among the first to recognize the presence of a lytic activity, later termed complement, capable of lysing bacteria. Among his contributions was the identification of endotoxin, now understood as the lipopolysaccharide component of outer membranes found on the surface of some bacteria (gram-negatives). Pfeiffer's bacillus, isolated from the lungs of victims of influenza, was long (mistakenly) thought to be the etiological agent of that disease. An argument can be made that it was Pfeiffer, not Almroth Wright, who should be credited with developing the first effective antityphoid vaccine (courtesy National Library of Medicine).

from time to time minute drops of the liquid be withdrawn in capillary tubes and examined microscopically, it is found that the vibrions, which were formerly, and in control animals which remain, actively motile, become in a very short time, under the influence of the serum, entirely motionless and later dead. They are first immobilized, then they become somewhat swollen and agglomerated [agglutinated] into balls or clumps....

Pfeiffer claimed that the reaction of the serum employed in this manner is so distinctly specific that it may serve for the differential diagnosis of the cholera-vibrion from other vibrions. If a mixture of the cultures of two vibrions is used in this experiment, only that species is destroyed which has been employed to immunize the animal whose serum is introduced with the cultures.[10]

Pfeiffer and his associate Wilhelm Kolle shortly afterwards applied this phenomenon in their proposal that immune serum could be used in the diagnosis not only of cholera, but also in differentiating typhoid infections from other intestinal infections; in part, these applications confirmed results which Gruber had previously reported.[11]

The authors [Pfeiffer and Kolle] say that by the aid of the serum of convalescents from typhoid fever, or of animals immunized against typhoid infection, typhoid bacilli can be differentiated from the bacillis coli communis and from other bacteria resembling the typhoid bacillus. This is accomplished by mixing the serum with cultures of the typhoid bacillus and introducing the mixture into the peritoneal cavity of guinea-pigs. A specific reaction appears, which can be followed microscopically. Agglomeration and agglutination of the bacilli occur, followed by deformity and final solution.... The bacteria belonging to the coli group, and all other similar bacteria, are not influenced in this test when the serum of animals immunized to the typhoid bacillus is employed. "This change takes place only with the typhoid bacilli, and is a specific reaction due to the bactericidal reaction of the typhoid serum."

It was further found, if the serum from a goat which had been immunized was diluted ... and a similar dilution made of the serum of non-immunized animals, and both solutions were then inoculated with a culture of the typhoid bacillus and placed in an incubator at 37°C, that after the expiration of one hour macroscopical differences in the culture could be observed, which increased in distinctness for four hours and then gradually disappeared. The reaction occurring may be described as follows: in the tube in which the typhoid culture is mixed with typhoid serum the bacilli are agglomerated in fine whitish flakes, which settle to the bottom of the tube, while the supernatant fluid is clear or only slightly cloudy. On the other hand, the tubes containing mixtures of bouillon with the cholera-serum, or the serum from non-immunized animals inoculated with the typhoid bacillus [control cultures], became and remained uniformly and intensely cloudy. These two serum-mixtures, examined microscopically in a hanging drop, also show distinct differences. The typhoid serum mixture inoculated with the typhoid bacilli exhibits the organisms entirely motion-less, lying clumped together in heaps; in the other mixture the bacilli are actively motile.

Pfeiffer and Kolle say further: "No such differences were shown when bacteria of the coli group were examined after mixture with the typhoid serum." They conclude: "*It would seem, therefore, that this method, which is of simple execution in any laboratory, may be of great practical value as an aid to differential diagnosis*"[12] [emphasis added].

Pfeiffer and Kolle clearly used Gruber's work as a precedent in describing an agglutination reaction in which substances in serum—antibodies in our contemporary understanding of the process—could be utilized not only for identification of the organism, but also explicitly stated that the pro-cedure could be used for diagnostic purposes.

Not everyone fully accepted Pfeiffer's and Kolle's conclusions as applied to identification of a range of organisms. Gruber in particular argued that the work described by the former with respect to the cholera bacillus (among Gruber's earlier accomplishments had been developing a method to differentiate among the vibrios) was lacking in specificity. How-ever, Gruber conceded the procedure was more applicable when applied to typhoid, concluding "that these investigations will render great assistance in the clinical diagnosis of cholera and typhoid fever."[13] Durham, building on more complete experimental data, was equally certain that the aggluti-nation reactions described by Pfeiffer and Kolle as well as his mentor Gru-ber could be applied in diagnostic tests. His report was based in part on his own research at Guy's Hospital in London, working in collaboration with Gruber in Vienna. The significant portions of the report are as fol-lows:

(1) A remarkable series of effects are produced on an emulsion of actively motile microbes by the addition of minute quantities of potent kinds of serum; (2) These effects have been observed with the cholera vibrio, a vari-ety of other vibrios, the *typhoid bacillus* [emphasis added], the *Bacillus coli communis*, and the *Bacillus pyocyaneus*…. (4) The most prominent of the effects thus produced consists of an immediate aggregation of the bacteria into clumps; this is combined with loss of motility. Marked inhibition of growth also occurs. (5) The formation of clumps can be detected readily by the naked eye. Eventually they gravitate to the bottom of the tube contain-ing them…. (8) The more intense the action of the serum, the more rapid and the more complete are the changes which ensue…. (10) Normal serum, and the serum obtained by immunizations with totally unrelated groups of organisms, do not interact upon the unrelated microbes…. (14) All the typhoid bacilli from nineteen different sources [sixteen sources as described in *Epitome*] hitherto observed react with typhoid serum; none of them react

with the *Bacillus coli* serum.... (16) The agreement in action of the typhoid
bacilli points to the use of the method for diagnostic purposes. Given a
young culture and typhoid serum, a diagnosis can be made in a few minutes.[14]

Durham also recognized limitations in what came to be known as the
Gruber-Widal test (eventually shortened to simply the Widal test). In
December 1896, following the respective reports of Grünbaum and Widal
on their own research into a diagnostic test (see below), Durham described
his use of the agglutination reaction in confirmation of suspected cases of
typhoid fever:

> Their observations [Grünbaum and Widal] have been made with the view
> of seeing whether the serum of individuals, healthy or suffering from other
> diseases, was endowed with an agglutinative power upon the typhoid bacil-
> lus. My own observations, which were commenced early last summer, were
> undertaken on other lines—namely, to see whether a positive reaction could
> be obtained in all cases of undoubted typhoid fever. It is clear that if posi-
> tive evidence is not obtainable in all instances the diagnosis cannot be
> absolutely fixed in cases of doubt. Dr. Grünbaum has shown that in cases of
> other than typhoid fever the blood serum has no positive effect upon the
> typhoid bacillus when it is sufficiently diluted; Dr. Widal's observations
> agree.... My observations upon typhoid fever in man show that positive
> results are not invariably obtainable, consequently some cases will remain
> doubtful even with this addition to the means of diagnosis. It is to be noted
> that all the cases in the following table were clinically typical cases of
> typhoid fever, and they therefore stand or fall together. The acuteness or
> mildness of the attack and the occurrence of relapses do not appear to be
> factors which necessarily conduce to the amount or presence of typhoid
> "agglutinins" in the serum.

Patient No.	Nature of Attack	Period When Tested	Reaction
1	Sharp single attack	During pyrexia, 14th day	None
2	"	Convalescent 16 days	None
3	"	During pyrexia, 3rd week	Well marked
4	Relapse after sharp attack	During pyrexia, 8th day of relapse	Moderate
5	"	Convalescent ten days	Fairly well marked
6	Sharp attack with relapse	Convalescent 18th day after relapse	None
7	Sharp attack, no relapse	Convalescent fourteen days	Fairly well marked

Patient No.	Nature of Attack	Period When Tested	Reaction
8	Mild attack followed by mild relapse	Convalescent seven days	No action
9	"	Convalescent ten days	Very well marked
10	Sharp attack, four relapses	Convalescent six weeks	Very well marked

Reaction Obtained with Serum from Typhoid Patients (Adapted from Durham)[15]

It will be observed in this table that the reaction is not always obtainable either during the original attack or during relapses or after them. The cases from which Observations 1 and 2 and 6 were taken were clinically typhoid fever without a shadow of a doubt. However, the study of the serums of immunized animals (rabbits, etc.) shows that they have little or no clumping action shortly after the first immunizing inoculation, and the typhoid fever patient or convalescent is really *only immunized to a very slight degree* [italics in original]—a degree, however, which is generally sufficient to protect him from further attacks....

It may be concluded that in recent cases of typhoid fever an absolute diagnosis cannot always be obtained by means of the serum test, but this means of diagnosis should not therefore be discarded, nor should it be allowed to fall into discredit by overrating its real value.[16]

Assuming of course that the three cases—30 percent of the subjects in this report—from which serum produced no visible reaction when mixed with the typhoid bacilli were indeed those of typhoid fever, a caveat for which Durham appears certain, it is unclear as to the reason for negative results. It should be kept in mind that these represented the earliest examples of the Widal test being used for diagnosis of the illness. William Welch, dean of the Johns Hopkins School of Medicine, in a later review of the subject, addressed the loss of agglutinative activity over time: "In the majority of cases the specific agglutinative power of the blood diminishes in the first weeks or months after cessation of the fever and disappears within a year. Exceptionally it may vanish as early as eight or ten days after the fever. Widal and Sicard noted its disappearance on the eighteenth and twenty-fourth days, Breuer on the seventeenth and twenty-fifth days, E. Fraenkel on the twenty-eighth day after defervescence, etc. *Disappearances at such early dates as these are, however, not the rule*"[17] [italics added]. An answer to why several examples shown by Durham above were reportedly negative for agglutinative activity must remain unknown.

Durham also, and perhaps inadvertently, alluded to a shortcoming of the (Widal) test as applied by Gruber as well as Pfeiffer and Kolle to convalescent patients. As pointed out by Sir Percival Horton-Smith (Hartley) in his Goulstonian lecture in March 1900, during which he discussed the early research carried out by Gruber and Durham, "The work of these observers had been done with the sera of animals already thoroughly immunized, and though Gruber was prepared to find the agglutinating properties present in the blood *after* [italics in original] an attack of typhoid fever it did not at first occur to him that the blood *during* [italics in original] the attack itself might also show the phenomenon. Here, then, was the opportunity of Widal, who on June 26th, 1896, announced the discovery that even during the disease itself the agglutinative power was present in the blood and that therefore the reaction served as a means of clinical as opposed to bacteriological diagnosis."[18] In his history of the subject Horton-Smith cited many of the significant researchers in that field, with the noted absence of Albert Grünbaum.

Neither Widal nor Grünbaum carried out their research in a so-called vacuum, if one may apply an old cliché. As described above, a significant background to the development of the diagnostic test was provided by the earlier work of others, most notably Gruber, Pfeiffer and Kolle. While these individuals were arguably the most notable contributors, by no means were they the only bacteriologists whose work was built upon by Widal and Grünbaum. Precedent for an agglutination reaction was demonstrated by Drs. Albert Charrin and Henri Roger in 1889 when they observed that blood obtained from vaccinated animals was capable of agglutinating the infecting bacteria:

> Our first investigations, pursued with Dr. Charrin, were made upon the bacillus pyocyaneus [now known as *Pseudomonas*]. Blood taken from normal and vaccinated animals was kept for twenty-four hours, when the serum was separated and put in tubes.... A very small dose ... of pyocyaneus culture, prepared in bouillon, was then introduced into the tubes, which were shaken and subjected to study. Some experimenters thought that the germicidal action of the serum under these conditions depended simply upon the fact that the culture made in bouillon was transferred to a different medium—i.e., the serum. We therefore often took our virus from cultures made in normal liquid serum. The results were identical in both instances. In fact, on the following day it was possible to clearly see with the naked eye notable differences in the mode and intensity of vegetation of the microbe, according as the culture was made in normal serum or in serum obtained from vaccinated animals. The normal serum was completely opaque, turbid, and of a bluish-green color. It contained a few flocculi which increased in number in the following days. On the other hand, the serum of the vaccinated animals became but very slightly turbid. The bacilli were united in small masses floating in the fluid. On the following days, the development was more noticeable, and the differences, although appreciable, were less striking.

When, however, the animal is well vaccinated, the cultures made in its serum always preserve a peculiar appearance. The fluid remains clear, and the microbes are united in small masses which are scattered when the tube is shaken.

Similar results were observed with the use of serum from animals vaccinated with other bacteria, including vibrio and the anthrax agent.[19] While the mechanism underlying the phenomenon observed by Charrin and Roger was unknown in 1889, it was increasingly obvious that substances in immune serum were capable of agglutinating or inactivating the organisms. Charrin and Roger had demonstrated their results in growing cultures of the respective organisms. However, in 1895 Belgian bacteriologist Jules Bordet, while working at the Pasteur Institute, observed that the results could be duplicated using serum from an immunized animal mixed with a culture which had already been grown.[20]

Albert Sidney Frankau Grünbaum (Leyton) (1869–1921)

Albert Sidney Frankau Grünbaum/Leyton is an almost forgotten figure in the development of the agglutination test for identification and diagnosis of typhoid fever. As noted earlier, his name was not even included among the researchers highlighted by Horton-Smith in his Goulstonian lecture on the history of the Widal test. Even though his surname was obviously German—more about that below—he was born in London, the son of Joseph Grünbaum, a merchant and naturalized British citizen, and Delia Frankau. Grünbaum graduated from Gonville and Caius College in Cambridge in 1891 with a degree in natural sciences, and an M.A. two years later, followed by his medical degree. He also became a member of the Royal College of Physicians of London. He carried out clinical work at St. Thomas's Hospital and Birmingham General Hospital. In 1896, working then in Vienna, he carried out the agglutination tests that arguably preceded those developed by Fernand Widal.

Following Grünbaum's election as FRCP in 1903 he was appointed director of cancer research at the University of Liverpool; that same year he delivered the Goulstonian lectures of the Royal College of Physicians of London, building on his own work in the area of agglutination reactions to present a contemporary history of "Theories of Immunity and Their Clinical Application." In his presentation Grünbaum extensively discussed and compared the "rival" theories of Metchnikoff's cellular theory with that of Paul Ehrlich's side-chain/humoral theory of immunity. In a prescient statement, Grünbaum suggested, "The two chief theories of the present day are those promulgated and supported by Metchnikoff and Ehrlich respectively. Originally opposed to one another, like the humoral and iatro-chemical theories of the Middle Ages, they are really only rays refracted at different angles from the same source of light, and will ultimately be made to fuse into one brilliant cellulo-humoral theory of immunity."[21] Grünbaum would ultimately be proven correct.

In 1904 Grünbaum joined the faculty of the University of Leeds, as a professor of pathology, where he subsequently became dean of the medical school. During the war he served as a consultant with the rank of major until ill health forced him to resign. British prejudice against anyone who sounded German or had a German surname, a situation which occurred as well in the United States, resulted in Grünbaum's changing his surname to Leyton in 1915, despite the fact he was a British citizen by birth. When he died in 1921, among the eulogies provided by Leyton's contemporaries which attested to his character was that of Sir Charles Sherrington, with whom Leyton had been associated at St. Thomas's Hospital:

> As one who knew Professor Leyton well and was intimately associated with him in some of the work which he did, may I add a word of tribute to his memory? None who had close contact with him could fail to be impressed by features of his thought and character which make his relatively early death an untimely loss to scientific medicine. He combined in rare measure enthusiasm for research with a critical, and indeed, highly self-critical, atti-tude of mind. An example earnest of his power of achievement was seen in his discovery of the agglutination reaction as a help to typhoid diagnosis, a discovery fraught with such high and still unexhausted consequences. Widely read and proficient, he was ever on the alert to take avail of means from the progress of collateral science for the immediate profit of medicine itself. He had imagination and at the same time no man endeavored more sincerely than he to control theoretical suppositions by observational data. The advance of practical medicine was with him a passion; in his devotion to that end he spared no labour or personal sacrifice. Though so much of his time and thought was given to laboratory work and technique, he was not one for whom these latter become per se the sole preoccupation. My recollection of him is of one for whom the interest of the laboratory was ancillary to and simply enhanced his interest in practical medicine. He was a man of high ideals, and to know him well was to realize the more his integrity of purpose, and his generous nature and the essential kindness of his heart.[22]

Both Grünbaum and Widal presented their respective work on the agglutination of typhoid bacilli using immune sera during the first half of 1896. However, Widal had begun this work some years earlier while working with André Chantemesse. In 1888 Chantemesse and Widal discovered that extracts prepared from typhoid bacilli, when injected into animals, were capable of providing a level of immunity.[23] They later found that if one injected guinea pigs with a combination of live typhoid bacilli and blood from a patient with typhoid fever the blood contained a "preventive power" which resulted in survival of the animal.[24] While this work was preliminary, it laid the groundwork for the application of an agglutination reaction in diagnosis of typhoid fever using the serum from a suspected patient.

André Chantemesse (1851–1919)

André Chantemesse was born in Le Puy-en-Velay, the son of a lace manufacturer. Until he was twenty-five years of age he worked in Paris in the lace industry, following which he enrolled in the Medical School of Paris. After a two-year medical training program he served as an *interne des hôpitaux* (a medical intern) until 1885. In 1884 he received his doctorate; his thesis involved the investigation of tubercular meningitis. In 1885 he spent a year working with Robert Koch in Berlin, learning techniques in the young field of bacteriology in a manner common among young physicians interested in research. Returning to Paris the following year, Chantemesse began a long collaboration with Fernand Widal in the study of typhoid fever; in 1888 he was awarded the Breant Prize from the French Academy of Sciences for their work with an infectious disease: typhoid fever. Among the accomplishments of Chantemesse in his collaboration with Widal was the demonstration "that the serum from animals vaccinated with the soluble products of cultures of Eberth's bacillus possesses

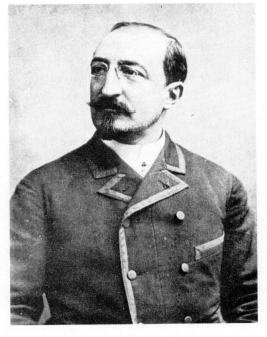

André Chantemesse (1851–1919), French bacteriologist who, in the 1880s with Fernand Widal, developed one of the first vaccines to be tested against typhoid fever (courtesy National Library of Medicine).

immunizing properties against the action of the virus, and that the same serum also possesses curative properties in experimental typhoid infection which is in process of evolution. The serum from an individual who has recovered from typhoid fever weeks, months and even years previously possesses preventative and therapeutic properties against experimental infection, while the serum of an individual who has not had typhoid fever is not, as a rule, endowed with the same power."[25] During Chantemesse's later professional career he was appointed professor of comparative and experimental pathology as a member of the faculty of medicine in Paris and a member of the French Academy of Medicine. His final years were spent as a member of the board of directors for the Pasteur Institute.

So the question of priority becomes not so much who developed the agglutination test using a mixture of immune serum and typhoid bacilli, but who reported a practical means to utilize the test. As described above, Gruber used the serum from patients who had already recovered from the illness. A method for diagnosis of typhoid fever in the patient had also been developed by this time. Developed independently by Albert Grünbaum at the Hygienic Institute in Vienna and Fernand Widal in Paris, this more important application of the test utilized serum from a patient suspected to be ill with the disease; this allowed a diagnostic use to be more practical. Thus Widal announced his discovery that year (1896).

> On June 26th last [1896] I brought before the Medical Society of the Paris Hospitals a new method—to which I gave the term "sero-diagnosis"—by which typhoid fever could be recognized almost instantaneously by simply observing microscopically how the serum of a patient acted on a culture of Eberth's bacillus. [On 26 June 1896 Widal had lectured at the Société Médicale des Hôpitaux de Paris on the diagnosis of typhoid fever using his agglutination procedure; typhoid patients from the Paris hospital had served as a source of serum.] I described several processes to establish the sero-diagnosis, some being slow and others rapid. Among the slow processes one consisted in adding a few drops of serum to a culture of Eberth's bacillus in bouillon already cloudy, and observing a few hours later whether the bouillon became clear again and if, at the same time, a precipitate was formed at the bottom of the tube. The other process consisted in adding to a tube of fresh bouillon a few drops of serum, then introducing into it a trace of a culture of Eberth's bacillus, and placing the tube in an oven at a temperature of 37°C, and observing whether after fifteen or twenty-four hours a precipitate had formed at the bottom of the tube, showing under the microscope heaps of microbes, leaving the bouillon almost completely clear....
>
> For ordinary daily practice I prefer the improvised process. I have shown that all that was necessary was to add a drop of serum or even a drop of blood taken from the tip of the finger of the patient to ten drops of a young

culture in bouillon of typhoid fever bacilli, and to see almost immediately under the microscope of "heaps" or agglomerations of bacilli, which often allows an almost instantaneous diagnosis of typhoid fever to be made. I ended my first communication by saying: "Here is a simple and rapid process which can be employed by everyone, necessitating no laboratory material. All that is necessary is to have at one's disposal pure cultures of Eberth's bacillus, a microscope, and a few drops of serum or even only one drop of the blood of a patient."

Widal further elaborated on the preliminary methods he had used to carry out his reaction as well as pointing out before whom he had presented this work.

On July 23rd and 31st at the Medical Society of the Paris Hospitals, and on July 29th in the *Presse Medicale*, and on August 6th at the Medical Congress of Nancy I took up this question alone and in collaboration with M. [Jean-Athanase] Sicard. We have shown that the reaction could be produced instantaneously if a pure culture of Eberth's bacillus on gelatin is diluted with pure bouillon and the suspected serum is immediately added. We have indicated that the reaction could be obtained with dried serum or dried blood coming from patients suffering from typhoid fever....

The agglutination of the microbes by the serum of immunized animals has been under consideration since 1889. As regards the infection of typhoid fever, we have stated previously that Pfeiffer and Koll had shown that the serum of animals rendered immune against the infection of typhoid fever as well as the serum of convalescents from typhoid fever, injected into the peritoneal cavity of a guinea-pig at the same time as a culture of Eberth's bacillus, possessed the property of rapidly immobilizing, of agglutinating, and deforming the microbe present in the serous cavity. We also mentioned that [Herbert Edward] Durham and [Max von] Gruber had previously shown that the serum of animals rendered immune against experimental typhoidal infection had the power of immobilizing and uniting in heaps or masses in vitro Eberth's bacilli in suspension in a liquid.[26]

Georges-Fernand Widal (1862–1929)

Georges-Fernand Widal was born in Dellys, Algeria, his father both an army surgeon and medical inspector of the army. Widal's uncle was Mathieu Hirtz, professor of pathological and clinical medicine, head of the clinic at the medical school and dean of the faculty of medicine in Strasbourg. Following his father's and uncle's profession, Widal studied medicine at the University of Paris. As an undergraduate he was awarded a position as Interne des Hôpitaux, assistant physician; he earned his doctorate by the age of twenty-six, his thesis dealing with the study of puerperal fever. He continued his studies of the etiological agent of that disease at Lariboisiere

Hospital in Paris, isolating what appeared to be chains of streptococci from a variety of illnesses in addition to puerperal fever, including erysipelas. Widal's conclusion was that the puerperal fever, often a postpartum killer of women, was associated with the bacterium *Streptococcus pyogenes*: "It is possible to produce in rabbits any type of infection with the same microbe, as has been proved by M. Widal in Professor [Victor André] Cornil's laboratory in Paris…. What effect this new discovery, that the same microbe produces infection both in surgical and in puerperal affections [*sic*] will have in regard to prevention and cure is yet to be seen, but many of our local scientists cannot believe that this agent is introduced either by the respiratory or by the alimentary tract, so that in the case of wounds and in the case of the uterus some local door of entrance must be left open by the surgeon or by the accoucheur [obstetrician]. It need hardly be added that strict antisepsis is the only practical indication to be drawn from these facts."[27]

Georges-Fernand Widal (1862–1929), French bacteriologist credited with development of the Widal test, a tool used for diagnosis of typhoid fever (courtesy National Library of Medicine).

During the two years he spent working in the laboratory of Professor Cornil, Widal taught a course in bacteriology while at the same time carrying out a collaboration with André Chantemesse in the study of pathogenesis of typhoid fever. It was during these years that he produced the preliminary work demonstrating the ability of immune sera to inactivate the typhoid bacillus. As described above, this work culminated in a diagnostic test for typhoid fever which Widal reported in the summer of 1896. Widal spent the latter half of his professional life in a variety of clinical and pathological studies. In 1904 he was appointed instructor in medicine at the University of Paris, and in 1911 became professor of pathology and internal medicine, a position he held until his death. During this time he also joined the staff of the Hospital Cochin in Paris, a hospital which specialized in providing care for the indigent. In a collaboration with the French physician Georges Hayem, in 1907 he described a form of hemolytic anemia, later to be known as Hayem-Widal Syndrome. At his death he was considered the standard-bearer of French medicine.

Working independently in Vienna, Albert Grünbaum reported at nearly the same time the results of his own agglutination test for identification of typhoid:

> If a drop of an emulsion of a motile pathogenic organism is mixed with the drop of the serum of an animal immunized against this particular bacillus the micro-organisms collect together in "clumps" and lose their mobility. The importance of this reaction, which had been seen by others, was first recognized and studied by Gruber and Durham. They threw out the suggestion that it might be made of diagnostic value in the sense that bacteria cultivated from the stools of cholera or typhoid fever patients might be identified by its aid. But it appeared likely on a priori grounds that the "agglutinins" found in the serum of immunized animals would also be formed in the human body during an attack of enteric fever or cholera (it being already known that "protective" substances [which we now recognize as antibodies], at any rate, are so formed); and at Professor Gruber's suggestion I undertook the investigation of this point as part of the question whether immunity and protection are not (in certain diseases) dependent on and proportional to the agglutinins present. The serum of normal guinea-pigs has rarely any pronounced agglutinative action, but it does not follow that the same would hold good for man, and an examination of some thirty cases of normal and diseased individuals … showed the presence of agglutinins in persons not suffering and not having suffered from enteric fever (or cholera). Although anticipating matters, it may be here stated that hitherto *it is only in cases of enteric fever that the serum shows a distinct agglutinative action within thirty minutes when diluted sixteen times* [italics in original], and hence this reaction can be used as a diagnostic sign. If the reaction occur in still greater dilution its diagnostic value is correspondingly increased…. [Grünbaum completes his report with a comment about Widal's observations.] Whilst this work was in progress a short communication by Widal applying a similar method macroscopically has been published in the *Semaine Médicale*. It requires, however, a larger quantity of blood and a longer time, and apparently, from the rather meagre description, a final resort to the microscope; and in one case, at any rate, I was unable to detect the reaction.[28]

In his own presentation of his work Widal responded to Grünbaum's final comments:

> Up to June 26th, 1896, the date of my first communication, the phenomenon of agglutination had been considered as a "reaction of immunity"

appearing only in immunized animals. I was the first to show that it was indeed a "reaction of infection," that it appeared in man during the first days of the disease, and I thus arrived at the conception of sero-diagnosis and its applications. A few days after my first communication, confirmative facts were presented by different clinicians and today some hundreds of observations of positive sero-diagnosis have already been published in Europe and America. Up to the present day my improvised process has almost always been preferred by experimenters. It is the same process which M. [Charles] Achard and M. [Raoul] Bensaude have employed for the sero-diagnosis of Asiatic cholera. I was, therefore, very much surprised to find an article on the Agglutinative Action of the Human Serum for the Diagnosis of Enteric Fever, published in the *Lancet* of September 19 last—that is, nearly three months after my first publication—by Dr. Grünbaum, who proposes a much more complicated process than my extemporaneous method, and only adds at the end of his article, as history of sero-diagnosis, the following: "Whilst this work was in progress a short communication by Widal applying a similar method macroscopically has been published in the *Semaine Medicale*. It requires, however, a large quantity of blood and a longer time and, apparently from the rather meagre description, a final resort to the microscope." If for a purely technical question Dr. Grünbaum, instead of being contented with an incomplete analysis given by a paper, had referred to the official text of my researches or to the *Presse Medicale*, which reproduced *in extensor* most of my works, he would have seen that I did not publish a *short communication* [italics in original] on the sero-diagnosis, but that since June 26th last I have published a series of articles on this subject, and that my favorite method is based only on microscopical examination, is extemporaneous and only necessitates a minimum quantity of blood. Dr. Grünbaum would have avoided an error which I desire to correct.[29]

Widal further included as a note the more recent application of his diagnostic technique:

I may add that in collaboration with M. Sicard I brought forward on September 29th at the Paris Academy of Medicine, and on October 9th and 16th at the Medical Society of the Paris Hospitals, new researches on sero-diagnosis and experimental and chemical researches on the agglutinative phenomenon which are too long to be considered here. I may also add that at present we have practiced sero-diagnosis in forty-five serious as well as mild cases of typhoid fever during its acute stage, and that we have searched for, without finding it, the agglutinative reaction of the blood of more than 200 individuals in good health or suffering from other diseases, by mixing the serum and culture of Eberth's bacillus in the proportions which I have indicated. The different authors who have controlled by researches have arrived at the same results.[30]

Several observations of scientific interest are apparent from this exchange. First, as Grünbaum correctly implied in the beginning of his report, Gruber and Durham's work utilized immune serum from sources which had recovered from the infection, and suggested a possible role for diagnostic use of the agglutination technique. And while Grünbaum had obviously carried out a significant preliminary study, the relatively small number of examples he used at the time were exceeded by the more extensive studies and detailed procedures either referred to by Widal or carried out on his own in Paris.

If anyone would have had claim to priority it would likely have been Max von Gruber, who had carried out his own preliminary studies several months earlier, even prior to that by either Widal or Grünbaum. Durham had returned to England by then and was out of the "equation," and Gruber waited until after Widal's report to publish his own results. This is why for a time the diagnostic technique was referred to as the Gruber-Widal reaction, eventually to be known simply as the Widal test.

Within a year most bacteriological laboratories—certainly the newer or larger ones—had adopted the Widal test for diagnosis of typhoid. The principle behind the test, agglutination of typhoid bacilli using serum from suspected patients, was further adapted. The original test involved the macroscopic observation of the reaction in a test tube; it required a significant amount of blood to be drawn from the patient. The refined version of the test could be carried out on what is now known as a depression slide. Only several drops of blood, sometimes acquired by bleeding the ear lobe, were required and the test could be carried out in a short period of time. It should be pointed out that this was largely the procedure described by Grünbaum in his September 1896 report in the *Lancet*: "A drop of blood is taken either from the ear or the finger … and the drop of serum blown out on to a glass slide.… The emulsion of typhoid bacilli is prepared by taking a small platinum loopful of a culture … and carefully rubbing it up against the side of a glass capsule.… A small drop of the diluted serum is then placed on a cover-glass, a drop as near as possible of the same size from the 'typhoid emulsion' mixed with it, the cover-glass placed on a vase-lined hollow slide, and the mixture examined as a hanging drop, with an immersion lens. Under the microscope it will be seen that the bacilli gradually form groups of three or four, which, by the addition of other bacilli, constantly increase in size until the majority are in 'clumps' with impaired or lost mobility."[31]

In addition to its diagnostic use, the test led to another discovery, that of the typhoid carrier. Carriers could be recovered patients (the bacterium was sometimes located in the gall bladder in some patients) or the person may have been completely asymptomatic. Typhoid Mary Mallon, or simply

Typhoid Mary, as she is known to history, would become the classic example of such a carrier.

The agglutination reaction would have applications in other areas of science as well. Karl Landsteiner, in his discovery and identification of blood groups, would apply the same reaction in determining iso-agglutinin antigens on human red blood cells.

9

Typhoid Carriers:
The Story of "Typhoid Mary"

Our studies have shown that all cases of typhoid of this type have arisen by contact, that is, carried directly from one person to another. There was no trace of a connection to drinking water.—Robert Koch[1]

As described in a previous chapter, identification and growth of the etiological agent of typhoid fever had been accomplished in the 1880s by associates of Robert Koch. The working hypothesis at the time was that if an individual had been exposed to the agent, one of two results would take place: either the person would develop the disease or the person's immune system would be sufficient to ward off the infection. Either way, the concept of an asymptomatic carrier was not immediately considered.

The first experimental evidence to suggest that typhoid infections could become chronic was reported in 1891. Arthur Blachstein from Johns Hopkins University injected rabbits with cultures of the bacillus typhi abdominalis (*Salmonella typhi*) and observed in about half the animals that typhoid bacilli could be isolated for as many as 15 weeks after the initial inoculation, even when the rabbits appeared healthy.[2] The bacilli seemed to be primarily present in the bile. The experiment was repeated a month later by William Welch, who confirmed that typhoid bacilli could be secreted in the bile of otherwise healthy rabbits up to four months after the initial inoculation.[3]

The significance of Blachstein's and Welch's observations was overlooked, and whether a similar chronic but asymptomatic infection would be possible in humans as well was not addressed in the report. However, within a few years other physicians did find similar results in humans— live typhoid bacilli could be isolated, sometimes even in the absence of actual illness. While at Johns Hopkins Hospital, Simon Flexner was able to isolate live, viable typhoid bacilli from the gall bladders of 50 percent of patients who had died from typhoid. Dr. G. Brown Miller, also at Johns Hopkins, was able to culture typhoid bacilli from a patient seven years after recovery. Dr. Harvey Cushing was able to isolate typhoid bacilli from a patient never known to have even had the disease.[4] In 1899 Dr. William Park, a member of the New York City Board of Health and later a key figure in the establishment of the first municipal diagnostic laboratory in the United States, suggested that similar chronic carriers of typhoid may "go about scattering infection which at any time may find conditions suitable for causing an epidemic of typhoid fever."[5]

In his Goulstonian lecture in 1900, Sir Percival Horton-Smith began to address in greater detail the possible role of the human carrier in transmission of the disease.[6] "The faeces are highly infectious at the commencement of the disease, and then later they become much less dangerous. How soon they become absolutely innocuous cannot be stated, but we must be prepared for the possibility of their remaining in some cases a source of danger for long periods after the patient is apparently well—as long, that is to say, as the bile continues to harbor the parasite."[7] Later in his lecture, Horton-Smith addressed the problem of chronic infection in greater detail, drawing on the earlier cited works of Blachstein and Welch:

> What is the length of time during which the bacillus may remain in the body? It was naturally supposed at first that as the fever passed away and as health returned the bacillus, the cause of the disease, would disappear from the tissues also. This apparently was demonstrated by the earlier observations. Thus it was shown long ago that if the spleen or mesenteric glands—the classical breeding grounds of the microbe—be examined late in the disease, no typhoid bacilli would be found, the organs being either sterile or possibly containing bacillus coli communis [*Escherichia coli*]. This has been noticed by [Simon] Flexner as early as the sixth week. Dr. [Emanuel] Klein recorded it in the ninth week, and recently a case dying at St. Bartholomew's Hospital in the thirteenth week showed the same disappearance of the specific organisms. The experiments of Blackstein [*sic*] and Welch, however, showed that, sometimes at least, the typhoid bacillus might remain for much longer times in the body. Thus after intravenous injections of the bacillus into rabbits, they found that the bile still contained the micro-organisms when the animals died or were killed at such long intervals as 84 days, 109 days, and even 128 days after the date of inoculation. The other organs were, however, found sterile.

These experimental results in animals naturally suggested that the same thing might occur in man after typhoid fever, and this has been amply proved, for we now know that it is nothing uncommon for the bacilli to remain dormant in the bile or the bone marrow for long periods, the patient, just like the experimentally inoculated animal, being meanwhile often in perfect health, and then, possibly after several years, under the influence of some passing stimulus, to resume their activity and to give rise now to periostitis [inflammation around the bone], now to osteomyelitis, or it may be to cholecystitis [inflammation of the gall bladder].[8]

After the turn of the century, it fell once again to Robert Koch to apply the observations of chronic infection by the typhoid bacillus as the source from which epidemics of the disease appeared. In the meantime, another significant advancement had been made by Koch's associates in isolation of the typhoid bacillus. In the decades since *Bacillus typhosa* had been isolated and demonstrated to be the etiological agent of the disease, its identification against a background of other organisms had remained a challenge. The bacillus could be grown easily enough on standard media, but so could other members of the flora. However, in 1902, Wilhelm von Drigalski and Heinrich Conradi from the Koch Institute developed the first selective medium useful in growing and identifying the organism. It allowed *Bacillus typhosus* to grow while at the same time inhibiting the background growth of other contaminating bacteria. The formulation, which contained aniline dyes such as crystal violet, would evolve into some of the most common selective and differential types of media such as eosin methylene blue (EMB) and MacConkey's agar, used in biological laboratories even a century later. The selective medium developed by Drigalski and Conradi found immediate use, as a small outbreak elsewhere in Germany was traced to four individuals with no symptoms of typhoid but from whose stool the bacilli could be isolated in stool samples.[9]

The first large-scale application of Drigalski's and Conradi's medium came about that same year following an outbreak of typhoid fever in the German city of Trier. A German commission, ostensibly under the auspices of Koch but placed in the charge of Paul Frosch, was sent to investigate the outbreak. Several years earlier, while working with Friedrich Loeffler, another of Koch's associates, Frosch was able to demonstrate that the etiological agent of foot and mouth disease was a filterable agent, a virus. This time, Frosch and members of the commission established that the source of this particular typhoid outbreak was drinking water contaminated with sewage. However, even with reinstitution of proper sanitation procedures, cases of typhoid continued to appear in surrounding areas. Koch concluded the source of the continued outbreaks was not sewage contamination, but rather healthy persons who were still excreting the agent. In a November 1902 address, Koch presented his hypothesis to a scientific

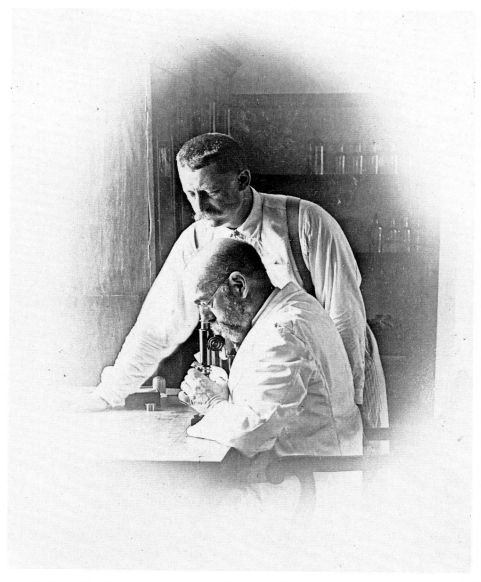

Richard Pfeiffer and Robert Koch (1843–1910). Koch, a German physician and bacteriologist, was among the most prominent scientists of his time. Koch himself was honored for his isolation of the etiological agents of diseases such as tuberculosis and cholera. He and his colleagues and associates have been credited with being among the most important figures in development of the Germ Theory of Disease. Koch was the first to propose that carriers might disseminate typhoid (courtesy Wellcome Library, London).

audience: "Our studies have shown that all cases of typhoid of this type have arisen by contact, that is, carried directly from one person to another. There was no trace of a connection to drinking water."[10]

In his address Koch suggested that a significant proportion of typhoid epidemics actually originated from seemingly healthy carriers. Consequently, both proper monitoring of persons possibly exposed to the agent and disinfection of excretions were critical in preventing outbreaks. The source of the typhoid agent in such excretions was well known by this time: the gall bladder. By the time of Koch's address, typhoid fever outbreaks had become so common in that region of southwest Germany that he recommended a monitoring station be established in Trier. Frosch was placed in charge. The success of that first station resulted in an additional ten experimental stations being set up during the following four years.[11] The major functions of the stations with their staffs of 35 were to examine and diagnose persons suspected of being infected with typhoid and to monitor any suspected carriers. In carrying out these tasks, the staffs' ability to isolate and identify the typhoid agents using the media developed by Drigalski and Conradi was of particular importance.

Several investigations led by associates of Koch lent credence to the possible role of carriers in dissemination of the disease. A possible outbreak in Berlin between October 1902 and June 1903 affected 122 persons. An investigation was carried out by Wilhelm Dönitz, who, after eliminating most cases as being either indeterminate or known origin, concluded that other sources of infection, such as direct contact, were possible.[12] Repeated outbreaks at Saarbrücken, where sanitation conditions were thought to be adequate, were attributed by Drigalski to healthy carriers.[13] Drigalski examined stool samples obtained from 64 cases of typhoid and found, even after convalescence periods of two months, typhoid bacilli could be isolated from seven of the individuals. One person continued to shed the organism as long as nine months later. Drigalski also was the first to isolate the bacillus from a healthy female carrier.[14] The observation that the carrier phenomenon might be more common than thought led Frosch to propose that typhoid bacilli may be able to lead a saprophytic (harmless) existence within the infected individual. Periodic excretion of the bacillus may have accounted for the intermittent outbreaks of disease even in the absence of evidence for sewage contamination. A summary of some of these earlier accounts was provided by the aforementioned William Park in a presentation before the American Medical Association, which was meeting in Chicago in 1908: "Levi and Kayser reported, in 1906, a case of a woman, 49 years old, who had had typhoid fever in 1903 and made a good recovery.

In 1906 the woman died from some other disease; autopsy was held nineteen hours after death. Typhoid bacilli were present in the liver, in the walls of the gall bladder and inside a number of calculi [gallstones]. Kayser reports that in Strassburg during the year[s] 1904–5, 13.5 percent of all cases of typhoid were traced to 6 of these typhoid carriers, all of whom were women and gave histories of having had typhoid from one to 27 years before."[15]

It was probable that the increase in proportion of carriers among convalescent patients actually reflected the greater use of the isolation medium developed by Drigalski and Conradi. The numbers were significant. Observations from a number of studies found that as many as 75–80 percent of typhoid cases examined during the third week were shedding the organism.[16] The length of time in which these individuals were secreting typhoid bacilli was determined. Samples were considered normal if they tested positive for fewer than ten weeks from the beginning of the illness. Patients who continued to excrete live bacilli for three months were arbitrarily considered as "temporary" carriers, while patients secreting for periods longer than that were considered "chronic" carriers. Since typhoid bacilli could also be isolated from individuals with no history of acute disease, the actual number of chronic carriers in the population was unknown.

Koch has been credited with acknowledging the carrier state of the typhoid bacillus, the first infectious agent to be recognized in that regard. Within a few years his hypothesis was confirmed not only by his associates at the Koch Institute, but also among physicians around the world. In most instances the bacillus survives in the gall bladder, and until the age of antibiotics treatment often involved cholecystectomy, the surgical removal of the gall bladder. Even in the 21st century, neither the surgical procedure nor antibiotic treatment is always successful in eliminating the bacteria.

The reason the organism may colonize and survive there remains unclear. Certain risk factors, such as the presence of gall stones or inflammation of the gall bladder, may contribute to the carrier state in some cases. The question of how the bacillus survives in a toxic environment of what in effect is a detergent also remains unknown. Studies have suggested that *Salmonella typhi* bacteria secrete a "bile-induced" biofilm which allows the organisms to survive on the surfaces of human gallstones.[17] Whether this would account for persistence in most carriers is unknown. While chronic carriers represent "no more" than 1–5 percent of recovered patients, as many as 25 percent of asymptomatic carriers have had no history of the disease.[18] Perhaps the most infamous of such historical chronic carriers was Mary Mallon, known more commonly as "Typhoid Mary."

The Story of Mary Mallon: Typhoid Mary

"Typhoid Mary" was one of many young, single Irish women who emigrated to the United States during the latter third of the 19th century, following on the heels of the tens of thousands who left during the potato famine of the 1840s. In the extensive biography written by Judith Leavitt, Mallon is described as being born in 1869, making her 15 when she arrived in the United States in 1883.[19] According to ancestry records, she arrived in June 1883 on board the ship *Ethiopia*, where her age is listed as 17, making her slightly older.[20] Regardless of her precise age, as with many such single women, she lived for a time with family in New York, in this case with an aunt and uncle, while she entered the servant workforce as a cook.

The first indication that Mallon may have been associated with outbreaks of typhoid occurred during the summer of 1906. She was working as a cook in the summer vacation home of New York banker Charles Henry Warren, a house he had rented from the George Thompson family. On August 27th, one of Warren's daughters developed typhoid fever. By September 3 another daughter, as well as Mrs. Warren, two maids and the gardener, had become ill with typhoid.

Knowing that with the lingering reputation of typhoid fever it would be difficult to rent the property in the future, the Thompsons hired several independent investigators in hopes of determining the source: Dr. Daniel D. Jackson, director of the laboratories of the New York City Department of Water Supply, Gas and Electricity, and Dr. E.E. Smith, a "well-known analytic expert."[21] Between September 12 and September 29, Jackson and Smith analyzed water samples from the faucets, storage tanks and the pump over the well. All were negative for typhoid bacilli. To test the possibility that sewage from the "water closet" might have leaked into the well water, Smith placed fluorescein in any sites which might have been a source of contamination: the water closet itself, cesspools, even in the stable manure vault. He found no evidence of leakage from these sites into the well water.

When the investigators hired by the Thompsons were unable to determine the source of the disease, during the winter of 1906 Thompson hired a civil engineer from New York named George Soper to investigate the outbreak. Soper was well known in this area of investigation, to the point that he was referred to as an "epidemic fighter." He had gained significant experience in the study of previous typhoid outbreaks, including earlier epidemics in places such as Ithaca and Watertown in New York, and in Butler, Pennsylvania. In the initial phase of his investigation he ruled out the most likely sources of the disease, including oysters from the local region, a sample of which had been brought to the house by "an old Indian woman." All sources were either negative or untenable. There were also no other reported cases in the area, the absence of which ruled out the possible source being the oysters. The only change in the routines carried out by the Warren family was that on August 4, prior to the outbreak, they had hired a new cook—Mary Mallon. Soper was at first skeptical as to whether a cook, especially one who likely would heat any food prior to serving, would be the probable source of the bacilli. However, it was also pointed out to him that in addition to any hot food with which Mallon might have been associated, she also prepared an ice cream dessert which included peaches, either of which could have been contaminated.

The obvious follow-up in Soper's investigation was to test stool samples from Mallon for the presence of typhoid bacilli. Unfortunately she was not readily available for testing, since she had left the Warrens' employ some time earlier. The next steps in Soper's investigation were twofold: backtrack Mary's employment record to determine whether the Warren outbreak was unique or merely the latest in a pattern, and locate Mallon herself for testing.

To be fair, Mallon may have understood, as did most persons in her place and time, that the spread of typhoid was associated with contaminated food and water. She would not have understood the concept of a typhoid carrier, someone who could be without symptoms and still be shedding the bacterium. In his memoirs, Soper himself acknowledged as much: "It will be remembered that in those days typhoid fever was far more common than it is today and that the knowledge of its transmission was less complete."[22] Some still attributed it to factors such as putrefying organic material or even sewer gas. In New York City, for example, 3,467 cases were reported in 1906, with 639 deaths. Lack of more complete testing meant it was likely these were only a portion of the total numbers for the city that year.[23]

With this in mind, it is a reasonable question to ask as to whether Soper himself was aware of the concept of typhoid carriers at the beginning of his investigation. At the very least, if and when he linked Mary Mallon with the Oyster Bay outbreak, this would provide the explanation for how she would transmit the disease, albeit unknowingly. It would appear he was indeed aware of chronic carriers. In his first extensive recounting of the completed investigation, read before the Biological Society of Washington, D.C., in April 1907, Soper stated, "We have here, in my judgment, a case of a chronic typhoid germ distributor, or, as the Germans say, a 'typhusbazillenträgerin [typhoid germ carrier].'"[24] Later statements made by Soper support the argument in favor of his knowledge of carriers at this time (see *n*24).

Soper was informed by Mrs. Warren that they had hired Mary Mallon through an employment agency called Mrs. Stricker's—likely "Mrs. R. Stricker and Nephew" located on 40 East 28th Street.[25] Other than noting that she did not appear particularly clean, Mrs. Warren could tell Soper little about her. Soper next went to the employment agency and obtained an employment history, comparing that history with reported cases of typhoid fever in the households where Mallon had worked. Between 1897 and 1907, at least eight families had employed the woman. Typhoid fever had broken out in seven of the families following her employment. Listed chronologically, those incidents were as follows.[26]

Mamaroneck, West Chester County, New York (Summer 1900)

A "young man" who visited with the family developed typhoid September 4, 1900, about ten days into the visit. Prior to his visit with the family, he had spent time at East Hampton on Long Island in the vicinity of an army camp at Montauk Point where fever had broken out. The initial belief was that he had been exposed while at East Hampton, possibly by drinking contaminated water. At the time, Mallon had worked for the family approximately three years with no signs of illness, either in Mallon or among the family. Whether she was the source of the illness in the man or whether he had previously been exposed remained uncertain. The ten-day interval would tend to rule out the latter.

New York City (Winter 1901–02)

Beginning in November, Mallon lived with a family approximately eleven months. On December 9 a laundress was admitted to Roosevelt Hospital. Dr. Robert J. Carlisle diagnosed her as suffering from typhoid fever. There was little follow-up investigation, and the source of the infection was never determined.

Dark Harbor, Maine (Summer 1902)

During the summer of 1902, the family of Coleman Drayton, a lawyer from New York, rented a home in Dark Harbor, Maine, shortly after hiring Mallon as a cook. The first case of typhoid fever among the household of nine—the footman—broke out on June 17. The following week a second case occurred, and by the time the initial outbreak was finished, seven of the nine were infected. Only Drayton himself, who had recovered from typhoid some years earlier and was presumably immune, and Mallon were spared. A trained nurse treating the family later became ill, as did a woman working there during the day. The outbreak was investigated by two physicians, Dr. Edwin A. Daniels of Boston and Dr. Louis Starr of Philadelphia, who believed the footman to be the source of the infection. Daniels initially thought the first three cases had represented simultaneous infection. But Soper ruled that out when he found no evidence they had eaten the same food or drunk from the same source of water. The two individuals spared the illness, Mallon and Drayton himself, took care of the sick to such an extent that after all had recovered, Drayton rewarded Mallon with a fifty dollar bonus—no small sum for the times.

Sands Point, Long Island
(Summer 1904)

During that summer, eleven members in the household of Henry Gilsey—the father in real estate and the son of the same name a lawyer—suffered an outbreak while in their summer home on Long Island. Mallon was hired on June 1, and one week later the laundress became ill with the disease. In subsequent days, the gardener, the butler's wife and the butler's wife's sister all became ill. The servants lived apart from the family, and while four of the seven servants became ill none of the family developed typhoid.[27]

Among those who investigated the outbreak was Dr. Robert Wilson, superintendent of hospitals for communicable diseases of the New York City Department of Health. Wilson believed the laundress might have been the source of infection, though he could find no evidence to support his contention.

Mallon was hired by a family at Tuxedo Park, New York.

Tuxedo Park, New York
(September–October 1906)

After leaving the employment of the Warren family, Mallon was hired as a cook by the George Kessler family, working there from September 21 to October 27. Fourteen days after Mallon's arrival, October 5th, the laundress became ill with typhoid. She was brought to St. Joseph's Hospital in Patterson, New Jersey, where she was treated by Dr. Edward C. Rushmore. Rushmore had not recalled a case of typhoid having appeared in Tuxedo

Park in recent memory. Other than Mallon, all servants had been employed for several years without incident.

New York City (Winter 1906–07)

Thus far, while at least twenty cases of typhoid fever might have been attributed to Mary Mallon, all had recovered. During November or December of 1906 Mallon was hired as a cook by an upscale Park Avenue family, that of Walter Bowen. A chambermaid became ill on January 23, 1907, and was brought to the Presbyterian Hospital in New York. A second victim, Bowen's daughter, died from typhoid on February 23, 1907, the first fatal case linked to Mallon.[28] It was here, in the kitchen of the Bowen household, that Soper finally caught up with Mallon and had a chance to talk with her.

By this time, Soper claimed to have identified twenty-six cases of typhoid associated with Mallon, including the newest victims, though only twenty-two were properly confirmed at the time. Fourteen were fellow domestic servants, while eight were members of the families which had hired her. This was actually a relatively small number against the backdrop of the time, in which 3,000 to 4,500 cases of typhoid fever were reported annually in New York City, but it was significant enough for Soper. In one respect he was caught in the thrill of the chase and perhaps even a promise of glory, feeling that Mallon's situation might make his career. Some of this might be inferred from comments made later in life following Mallon's death in 1938. In two letters quoted by Leavitt, Soper stated that while the media made reference to his work in the investigation, these same accounts "rob me of whatever credit belongs to the discovery of the first typhoid carrier to be found in America.... Suffice it to say I did not stumble upon her in the course of routine duties ... or as a blind disciple of Robert Koch. I was at the time a thoroughly trained and experienced epidemic fighter who had seen service in the laboratory and the field.... It was a difficult investigation."[29] But that would all come later. What came of his first interview with the woman? His first impression, recounted after her death, was considerably less than flattering:

> I first saw Mary Mallon thirty-two years ago, that is, in 1907. She was then about forty years of age and at the height of her physical and mental faculties. She was five feet six inches tall, a blond with clear blue eyes, a healthy color and a somewhat determined mouth and jaw. Mary had a good figure and might have been called athletic had she not been a little too heavy. She prided herself on her strength and endurance, and at that time and for many years thereafter never spared herself in the exercise of it. Nothing was so distinctive about her as her walk, unless it was her mind. The two had a

peculiarity in common. Those who knew her best in the long years of her custody said Mary walked more like a man than a woman and that her mind had a distinctly masculine character, also.[30]

One wonders whether Soper might have described a man in such terms. Whatever specific words Soper might have used during their first meeting were never recorded, but Mallon's response was unmistakable: "I [Soper] was as diplomatic as possible, but I had to say I suspected her of making people sick and that I wanted specimens of her urine, feces and blood. It did not take Mary long to react to this suggestion. She seized a carving fork and advanced in my direction. I passed rapidly down the long narrow hall, through the tall iron gate, out through the area and so to the sidewalk. I felt rather lucky to escape."[31]

Soper acknowledged that, in his mind, it was not critical that he obtain a fecal specimen to link Mallon with the outbreaks. The epidemiological evidence—the fact that typhoid appeared to follow in the wake of her employment—would appear to have been sufficient. Mallon's later response—that she was in perfect health with no evidence of infection and that with typhoid so common in the city the source could have been seemingly any-where—was hard to dispute on the surface. At that stage of the investiga-tion one could not completely rule out her contention. What Soper was accusing her of doing, spreading an epidemic which had now resulted in at least one death, was also incomprehensible to a woman with no medical training.

It would require a true undertaking to obtain definitive evidence, and time was not then on Soper's side. Once Mallon left the Park Avenue employment she could disappear among the masses anywhere in the city. Soper learned she often spent evenings in a Third Avenue rooming house with a "disreputable looking man who had a room on the top floor and to whom she was taking food."[32] After becoming acquainted with the man, Soper was allowed to see the room, a "place of dirt," occupied as well by a large dog.[33] Along with a friend, Dr. B. Raymond Hoobler, Soper con-fronted Mallon and once again was met with denial and a significant degree of anger.[34] Soper attempted to explain the circumstances, that he believes Mallon was the source of the infections in the households which had employed her. As if that accusation was not bad enough, his request that she provide fecal samples for testing was even more insulting in her mind. Soper and Hoobler left, "followed by a volley of imprecations from the head of the stairs."[35] One may safely assume these were not invitations to come back for another visit.

Because of the growing seriousness of the situation, and the potential difficulty of locating her once she changed employment, Soper brought the case before commissioner of health Thomas Darlington and Dr. Hermann Biggs, medical officer of the New York City Health Department, of whom he requested Mary Mallon be taken into custody for a more thorough examination, so it could be determined once and for all whether she was a carrier. In response, the department sent an inspector, Dr. Sara Josephine Baker, in an attempt to reason with Mallon. Baker, who a year later would become the first director of the New York City Bureau of Child Hygiene, had no greater success than had Soper earlier: "Mary slammed the door in her face."[36]

It was clear that Mallon could not be persuaded to cooperate. The next morning, March 20, Baker and three New York City police officers appeared at the door. When Mary realized who was there and what they intended, she ran back through the house and temporarily disappeared. Following footprints in the snow on the back of the property, the police officers eventually located Mallon hiding in a closet on an adjacent lot. As Baker later described the scene, "I told the policeman to pick her up and put her in the ambulance.... The ride down to the [Willard Parker] hospital was quite a wild one."[37] At one point during the ride, Baker was even forced to sit on Mallon. Given Soper's description of the strength of the angry woman, one can visualize a caged wildcat.

Fecal samples were obtained and examined in the laboratory of Dr. William Park three times a week between the date of her hospitalization, March 20, and November 16. In most of these samples they observed the presence of *Bacillus typhosus*, the agent of typhoid. The conclusion was inescapable: she was a typhoid carrier. Because she was likely to try to flee, Mallon was placed in an isolation ward at the hospital, which is where Soper visited her shortly afterwards.

As Soper later recounted the story, he again attempted to reason with her and explain the situation. She was a carrier, despite her seemingly healthy appearance, and whenever she went to the toilet the typhoid germs would contaminate her fingers. The implication here was she was not sufficiently washing her hands, one more accusation thrown at an obviously proud woman. It was well known by the first decade of the twentieth century that the typhoid bacillus was frequently maintained in the gall bladder. Soper suggested surgery to remove that organ in hopes of curing her carrier state. He even offered to write a book about the case, with Mallon receiving a portion of any profits, if she only would change her vocation. Mallon remained silent through the entire visit, then simply disappeared into the bathroom.

Mary remained in isolation for nearly three years, after which the health department agreed to allow her release on condition that she no longer serve as a food handler and that she report to the department on a regular basis. Despite having agreed to the demands of the health department, Mallon changed her name, sometimes being known as Marie Breshof, or simply Mrs. Brown. She also continued to work as a cook in a variety of places: restaurants, hotels, even a sanatorium in New Jersey. Wherever she worked, typhoid followed.

It was during this period that the name "Typhoid Mary" was coined. During the annual meeting of the American Medical Association in Chicago during June 1908, William Park presented a paper on the subject of typhoid carriers. This presentation included the story of a cook in the city who was a known carrier: "On March 20, 1907, a cook was brought to the laboratory to have the feces and urine examined. The history as developed by Soper revealed the fact that during the past eight years she had been employed in eight families and in seven of these typhoid fever had broken out within a few weeks or months of her arrival. In all, twenty-six cases and one death occurred. Just before her removal to the Department of Health two cases had developed in the [Bowen] family where she resided and one patient died. Bacteriologic examination revealed the fact that fully 30 percent of all the bacteria voided with the feces were typhoid bacilli.... A curious feature of the case is that the woman denies that she ever had typhoid fever."[38] As pointed out by Leavitt, Park identified the woman simply as a "cook," avoiding any form of public "outing" of Mallon.[39] At the time of Park's presentation, Mallon was in the hospital under isolation and seemingly posed no threat to the public. It was during the discussion which followed that the new term Typhoid Mary entered the professional lexicon. Park was apparently absent for the discussion.

Dr. William Litterer, a professor of histology, pathology and bacteriology at the Vanderbilt University School of Medicine, described a patient, a recent victim of typhoid fever, who had presented with post-typhoid necrosis of a rib. Upon culturing a sample of isolated pus months after the patient had recovered from the illness, Litterer observed large numbers of typhoid bacilli. The patient was treated with an autogenous vaccine prepared from the material and appeared to be recovering. In the context of treating chronic carriers, Litterer suggested that such a vaccine might be as useful as surgical removal of the gall bladder—Park's suggestion for a treatment.

Dr. Milton Rosenau, director of the Hygienic Laboratory in Washington, D.C., continued with the discussion: "I can not take Dr. Park's place, but feel sure that if he were here he would say that '*typhoid Mary*' [emphasis added] refuses to submit to surgical interference. She is perhaps justified in this conclusion, because the gall bladder is not the only source of the typhoid bacilli that appear in the feces. Surgical interference therefore may not always correct the condition. Sometimes the feces of these carriers contain such large numbers of typhoid bacilli as almost to displace the colon bacillus; it seems that the typhoid bacillus may take up a natural habitat somewhere in the intestinal tract independent of the gall bladder."[40]

An article in the William Randolph Hearst newspaper *New York American* on June 20, 1909, brought the name Mary Mallon before the general public, linking it to the nickname "Typhoid Mary." Mallon was still a relatively young woman in her forties when released from the hospital. But since most wealthy families utilized the same employment agencies as a source of servants, including those who were cooks, it was nearly impossible for Mallon to find long-term employment. As a result she frequently moved among a variety of low-paying positions, often infecting household members with the disease. Mallon even found employment at a maternity hospital where, ironically, they were carrying out tests on the efficacy of a typhoid vaccine.

The situation was again brought to Soper's attention, and after the New York City Health Department was notified, Mallon was placed in a house near the hospital on North Brother Island in the East River. The site had been established in the 1850s for the isolation of smallpox patients but had since been expanded to include other infectious diseases. Mallon spent over two decades there, working in the hospital and making occasional trips back to the city. Other than the incarceration, Mallon lived relatively peacefully until her death in 1938.

According to Emma [Goldberg] Sherman, a young technician who had a laboratory on North Brother Island and who employed Mallon during the 1930s, Mallon never accepted the reality that she was a carrier of typhoid: "She [Mallon] said the health officials didn't know what they were talking about and that they picked on her and that there was nothing wrong with her. That's the way she put it, that they picked on her and that she was healthy and how could she make people sick when she's healthy.... She denied it to her teeth."[41] The precise number of cases linked to Mallon is unknown. Soper attributed fifty-three cases and three deaths, though the actual incidence is likely significantly greater.[42]

George Soper

While George Soper is remembered primarily for his work in tracking the source of typhoid outbreaks in New York City and subsequently linking them to the cook named Mary Mallon, his professional career encompassed a range of areas. Born in 1870 in Southampton on Long Island, he earned a bachelor of science degree from Rensselaer Polytechnic Institute in Troy, New York, and a doctorate from Columbia University in 1899. His first professional job was that of civil engineer with the Boston Water Works, for which he worked in the field of sanitation. He subsequently was employed as a sanitation engineer with the Cumberland Manufacturing Company, then a manufacturer of filtration materials. When a devastating hurricane destroyed much of the city of Galveston, Texas, in 1900, Soper was placed in charge of rebuilding the sanitation and freshwater stations. In part as a result of his successful reconstruction of the systems, in 1902 Soper was appointed chief sanitary engineer of the New York City Department of Health.

It was in this role that Soper was requested by the state department of health in 1904 to investigate an outbreak of typhoid fever in Ithaca, New York, that had taken place the preceding year. Between January 1 and April 1, a total of 703 cases were reported to authorities; the actual number was probably greater, with estimates as high as 1,350. Since the population of the city was only slightly greater than 13,000, this meant 10 percent of the population likely became ill. There were 82 deaths.[43] Soper observed numerous possible sources of pollution of the water supply. One example in particular was that of a hotel which housed "people in search of health," some of whom may have been carriers of typhoid. In addition, heavy precipitation the previous December had washed a significant amount of filth into the water, which might have contributed to the outbreak.

Under Soper's supervision, the Ithaca Board of Health carried out inspections of over 1,300 wells which supplied water, as well as an equal number of "privies" which might have contributed to the problem. Water mains were flushed, sewage was collected—over 418,000 gallons—and refuse was burned.[44] Improvements in sanitation suggested by Soper were implemented in addition to changes carried out by the city on its own initiative that together ultimately controlled and ended the outbreak. Soper's reputation as a disease fighter grew with the successful investigation of the Ithaca outbreak, and he was called upon to investigate similar epidemics in other cities. It was in this capacity that he was requested in 1906 to investigate the outbreak in the Warren household on Oyster Bay, during which he implicated Mary Mallon as the source.

Still a young man after completing his role in the story of Typhoid Mary, Soper was hired by the New York Transit Commission to investigate the ventilation system in the New York subway system which had recently been finished. Drawing upon his expertise as an engineer, Soper carried out an extensive comparison with analogous systems utilized in other cities such as Boston and London in providing recommendations pertaining to the intake and exhaust of fresh air.[45] Over 5,000 analyses were carried out, and many of his recommendations were subsequently implemented.[46]

Soper was later appointed as a commissioner of the Metropolitan Sewerage Commission, on which he served as president of the scientific works bureau. His duties included the oversight of sewage disposal in the city. In 1914 he was hired by the city of Chicago to oversee similar sanitation procedures. Following the entrance of the United States into World War I, Soper served as a major in the Sanitary Corps of the army. During his tenure in this position he provided epidemiological data pertaining to the influenza outbreak in 1918 as well as a very vivid description of the acute illness: "The onset is sudden. The patient can often tell the exact moment of his attack. In the typical case he is very sick—wholly incapacitated for exertion. He lies curled up and can hardly be aroused for food."[47]

In 1923 Soper became managing director of the American Society for the Control of Cancer, the forerunner of the American Cancer Society. He retired from that position after five years but continued to serve as a consultant for the organization. As a member of the American Society of Civil Engineers, Soper spent a portion of his later years traveling through foreign cities and providing advice in sanitation procedures. In many instances he found methods of disposal in foreign cities to be superior to those methods used in New York City. Some of the changes he recommended for New York were eventually implemented. Illness and advancing age eventually limited his ability to serve in similar capacities, and he died in 1948.

10

Vaccination as a Preventive Measure: The Work of Sir Almroth Wright and Beyond

Who could deny the triumphs of anesthetics, antiseptic surgery, and vaccination, even in a world burdened with human short-coming and sin.—William Osler[1]

Vaccination as a means of protection against disease had been practiced as far back as the 1790s, when British country physician Edward Jenner tested the belief that inoculation with pus from the relatively mild disease of cowpox could provide immunity against smallpox. Initial implementation of the procedure generated no shortage of controversy. But one could not argue with success, and 100 years later most scientists accepted the validity of the process even if its mechanism remained somewhat obscure.

The French and German schools of scientific thought remained advocates, respectively, of either a cellular or a humoral basis (see Chapter 8). It was the French school, led largely by the theories and practice of chemist Louis Pasteur, which developed many of the vaccines subsequent to the work of Jenner. While the term vaccination was coined by Jenner, from the Latin *vacca* (cow), since the first vaccine originated from an infection in that animal, it was Pasteur who applied that term to immunization against other diseases. During the first years of the 1880s, using attenuated etiological agents, Pasteur developed vaccines against several human and non-human animal diseases, including chicken cholera, anthrax, and, most notably, rabies.

Pasteur's methodology demonstrated that vaccine development was practical in providing immunization against a variety of diseases. Not only could inactivated bacteria function as immunological agents, but with the discovery of bacterial toxins it was determined that inactivated forms of these proteins could also serve to immunize, first nonhuman animals and then human beings, against disease.

It was initially unclear whether chemically-killed or heat-killed organisms could provide the same level of immunity as natural infections. Later in the 1880s, however, Daniel Salmon and Theobald Smith, scientists working in the United States Department of Agriculture, demonstrated that the etiological agent of hog cholera, when injected into pigeons, still provided immunity against the disease even after being heat-killed. The reasoning behind their experiments was a relatively straightforward application of the prevailing theories of immunity, ca. 1886:

> The nature of [such] acquired immunity has long been an interesting subject for speculation, and until comparatively recent times it has long been mysterious and incomprehensible. Since the demonstration of the germ theory of disease, it became evident that there were three possible explanations of it.
>
> 1. Something had been deposited in the body during the attack of the disease that was unfavorable to the specific germ.
>
> 2. Something had been exhausted which had been essential to the development of this germ.
>
> 3. The living tissues had acquired such a tolerance for the germ or for a poison which it produces, that they were no longer affected by it.
>
> If either the first or the third of these explanations were correct, it would appear possible that immunity might be granted by introducing into the tissues the liquids in which the specific germs had been cultivated and from which they had been removed by filtration [as would be the situation with toxins], or in which they had been killed by suitable methods. I have long been convinced of the correctness of this supposition, but it is only recently that I have been able to make a satisfactory demonstration of the principle.
>
> In these experiments I have used the virus of the contagious fever of hogs known as swine plague. This virus, cultivated in the laboratory in suitable liquids, is very destructive to pigeons when injected hypodermically in the region of the pectoral muscles, in doses of three-fourths of a cubic centimeter. To test the protective effect of the product of bacterial growth, the virus referred to was cultivated in a one percent solution of peptone. After a number of days' cultivation, the culture was raised to 58° to 60° centigrade, a temperature which soon kills the microbe; but to make sure that all life was destroyed, we invariably transferred a few drops of the heated liquid to a fresh tube of culture fluid. If any multiplication of the germs occurred, it was of course evident that the temperature had not been high enough or

was not maintained for a sufficient time. This made it necessary to repeat the operation.

Salmon carried out at least nine experiments in which he inoculated pigeons with the inactivated—heat-killed—organisms and tested their resistance when exposed to the wild-type agent. Of the nineteen pigeons thus immunized, eighteen were completely immunized, while the remaining pigeon recovered from the illness. Among the eight unimmunized controls, seven died from the infection. In a separate experiment the infectious agent was evaporated over a boiling water-bath and tested on two pigeons; one was successfully immunized.[2] The significance of Salmon's experiments lay in the demonstration that the heat-inactivated agent could serve to immunize an animal against disease; one need no longer rely on an attenuated but still living agent as the basis for the vaccine. As described in the preface for this book, Salmon and Smith mistakenly ascribed the eponymously named *Salmonella* as the etiological agent. It was only some ninety years later that the agent was found to actually be a virus.[3]

During the years following Salmon's work significant progress was made towards control of several heretofore life-threatening diseases. Vaccines were developed against diphtheria and tetanus toxins by Kitasato Shibasaburo and Emil von Behring (1890) and against the cholera bacillus by Waldemar Haffkine (1892). It was during this period and against this background that Sir Almroth Wright first provided his contribution in the form of a vaccine against typhoid fever.

As described below in the brief biography of Wright, during September 1892 he joined the medical school associated with the Army Medical Hospital in Netley, located near Southampton in England. The hospital, known formally as the Royal Victoria Hospital, had been established during the 1850s as a result of the appalling sanitary conditions evident during the Crimean War; the medical school was incorporated several years later. Wright's duties as professor of pathology included teaching several mornings each week while at the same time establishing his own research program.

Wright's research at the time of his appointment consisted of parallel studies in blood coagulation and in the problem of coagulation of cow's milk when used as a substitute for human milk in nursing infants. Wright observed that the milk coagulation problem was often due to excess calcium in the cow's milk. If one treated the milk with a chelating agent, sodium citrate, the problem would be resolved: "The fact [is] that obstinate infantile constipation will often (I speak ... from a very small experience) disappear when the child is put upon a diet of citrated milk (i.e., milk which has been deprived of its excess of lime salts by an addition of 1–400th of citrate of sodium)."[4] The reverse was also applicable. Excessive hemorrhaging often resulted from minor wounds, and even in some cases following injection of either diphtheria antitoxin or the anti-cholera vaccine developed by Haffkine. Wright found that administration of oral doses of calcium chloride appeared to contribute to blood coagulation. This alleviated the problem of "serous hemorrhaging," i.e., hemorrhaging into tissue. Conjecture that similar treatments might be useful in treatment of "boils, of croupous pneumonia, and of some cases of phthisis [tuberculosis] with considerable expectoration"[5] would prove unfounded. The same publication in the 1896 issue of the *Lancet* was significant for another reason: Wright referred to vaccination of both a horse and an officer in the Indian Medical Service [initials M.D.] with a prototype typhoid vaccine, albeit in the context of demonstrating the effectiveness of calcium chloride in controlling hemorrhaging. Each animal—human and nonhuman—was first immunized with dead typhoid bacilli, followed several weeks later with exposure to live virulent cells. A second officer [J.S.] received a culture of dead bacilli identical to that of the first officer. Neither horse nor human appeared to suffer ill effects.

The timing of Wright's work is important in determining who should receive proper credit in production of the first effective typhoid vaccine.[6] Though development of the first effective vaccine has been generally attributed to Wright, it is clear that some of the initial background work in immunization against this specific disease had already been carried out by the time of Wright's report. In 1886 Wasilij Sirotinin tested killed typhoid bacilli in rabbits and guinea pigs for possible toxic effects.[7] That same year the bacteriologist Eugen Fraenkel and his colleague, pathologist Morris Simmonds, inoculated animals with the bacillus, observing that approximately half of the animals developed what appeared to be typhoid. Interestingly, the authors also suggested that heating of the organisms might potentially inactivate them while still allowing them to retain the ability to serve as a vaccine.[8] Other investigators, including André Chantemesse and Widal, Ludwig Brieger, Shibasaburo and August Paul von Wassermann, reported similar results in their experiments: even the products of the typhoid bacilli were able to produce pathological changes and death. Whether these were the results of actual replication of organisms or toxicity associated with bacterial endotoxin, at that time poorly characterized, is unclear. Nevertheless, these same investigators found that serum from those animals in which immunization proved to be successful would indeed provide protection when injected into mice or guinea pigs subsequently exposed to virulent bacilli.[9]

In what may have been one of the first attempts to treat typhoid patients with this method, Eugen Fraenkel inoculated fifty-seven patients suffering from the disease with a heat-killed suspension of typhoid bacilli during the Hamburg outbreak in April 1893, ironically the same year in which that city established a treatment plant for chlorination of drinking water.[10] The treatment appeared to show some success, but the variability in severity of the disease made it difficult to accurately determine its efficacy. However, another feature of immune serum observed by those attempting to develop an effective vaccine. As described in an earlier chapter, studies carried out independently by Richard Pfeiffer, Wilhelm Kolle, Max von Gruber, Herbert Durham and even Fernand Widal during these years had demonstrated that immune serum from typhoid patients, when mixed with typhoid bacilli, could agglutinate the cells. While the underlying purpose of their work was for diagnostic purposes, it was not lost on these individuals that the same principle could be more widely applied in vaccine production.

An initial question dealt with how effective immune serum would be in protecting humans against the disease. Fraenkel's work showed promise. The principle certainly worked in nonhuman animals. As noted above, Brieger, Shibasaburo and Wassermann demonstrated that serum from immunized

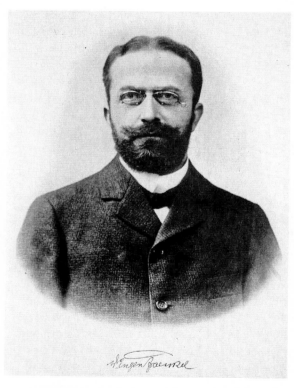

Eugen Fraenkel (1853–1925), German physician and bacteriologist who carried out initial attempts to treat typhoid patients with a heat-killed version of the bacillus in the 1890s (courtesy Wellcome Library, London).

animals was capable of protecting guinea pigs from the disease following intradermal injection. R. Stern observed similar results when using the serum from typhoid patients; injection of such "immune" serum would provide protection in mice, though he was less successful in immunizing guinea pigs.[11] Chantemesse and Widal likewise found that serum from typhoid patients would immunize animals against the disease. In one example, the serum demonstrated a protective effect in animals twenty years after the patient had recovered from the disease. The patient's serum was capable of protecting not only rabbits, but guinea pigs as well, against challenge with live bacilli, contrary to the results reported by Stern. The obvious control, serum obtained from individuals who had not been infected with the typhoid bacillus, showed no degree of protection. The reciprocal experiment, injection of serum from immunized animals into typhoid patients, showed no therapeutic effect.[12]

Wright and David Semple, a British army officer assigned to the Indian Medical Service, carried out the work which ultimately led to publication of their vaccine paper during the summer of 1896. As described briefly above, in his publication in an issue of the *Lancet* dated September 19, 1896 (see Ref. 4) Wright reportedly tested a prototype typhoid vaccine on two army officers. The results of a more extensive testing of the vaccine were reported the following January; it is this publication which is often considered to be the first description of the efficacy of a typhoid vaccine.[13]

The principle applied by Wright and Semple in development of the typhoid vaccine was clearly influenced by the prior work of Waldemar Haffkine, who produced a vaccine directed against cholera.[14] Wright and Semple acknowledged Haffkine's role in the opening paragraph of their report: "Mr. Haffkine suggested rather more than twelve months ago to one of us that the method of vaccination which has proved so effectual in combating cholera epidemics in India might, *mutatis mutandis*, be applied also to the prophylaxis of typhoid fever. Since that time, this question has been constantly engaging our attention, and we have gradually elaborated the method of antityphoid vaccination, which is to be briefly described in this paper."[15]

Haffkine's work provided the basis for Wright and Semple's subsequent study. But when did Haffkine and Wright, presumably, actually meet? "Rather more than twelve months ago" might suggest early the previous year. Perhaps this time period could be narrowed. While visiting Wright's laboratory at Netley early in 1893, prior to his departure for India where he would test his cholera vaccine, Haffkine demonstrated his procedure for preparing and testing the vaccine in animals. At the time, Wright was working with David Bruce in development of a vaccine against brucellosis, often known as Malta fever, who some years later would actually test a brucellosis vaccine on himself, with less than ideal results. Following Haffkine's departure, Wright and Bruce described Haffkine's anticholera vaccine in a publication for the *British Medical Journal*.[16] The anticholera vaccine used to treat three guinea pigs in Haffkine's demonstration was prepared by treating live "exalted" (virulent) cultures of the cholera bacillus with carbolic acid, a procedure at variance with that later used by Wright and Semple but one which still maintained the antigenicity of the culture. The success of the anti-cholera vaccine in part resolved the question of whether a culture of killed organisms would still function as a vaccine.

Haffkine arrived in India in March 1893, remaining in that country until September 1895, when he developed malaria, necessitating his return to England. He subsequently recovered, and on December 18, 1895, he presented the results of his vaccination work before the Royal College of Physicians of London and the Royal College of Surgeons of England.[17] It was likely during this period, December or January, that Wright had the opportunity to discuss Haffkine's work and develop procedures for more thorough testing of a typhoid vaccine. Building upon the precedent carried out by others, Wright and Semple first described the principles of their technique, followed by the thought processes which led to their final decision:

> The object of all vaccination processes is, first, to achieve a degree of immunity which shall be equal or greater to that which accrues to a patient who undergoes and recovers from an actual attack of the disease; and, secondly, to achieve that immunity without any risk to life or health.
>
> The first of these objects can, as far as is known, only be satisfactorily achieved by inoculating the patient with the micro-organisms (or the products of the micro-organisms) of the particular disease. The second object can be achieved in several ways. We may either, as in the Jennerian vaccination against small-pox, inoculate the patient with micro-organisms which have lost their virulence for man by being passed through a whole series of appropriately chosen animals. Or we may, as in the Pasteurian method of vaccinating against anthrax, employ in our inoculations artificially attenuated micro-organisms. Or, lastly, we may inoculate the patient with measured quantities of dead, but still poisonous, micro-organisms.
>
> It is this last method which we have adopted in the case of our typhoid vaccinations. The advantages which are associated with the use of such dead vaccines are, first, that there is absolutely no risk of producing actual typhoid fever by our inoculations; secondly, that the vaccines may be handled and distributed through the post without incurring any risk of disseminating the germs of the disease; thirdly, that dead vaccines are probably less subject to undergo alterations in their strength than living vaccines [that is,

since the organisms were no longer replicating it would be easier to calculate a consistent dose of cells for the vaccine].[18]

Instead of treating live cultures of typhoid bacilli with carbolic acid, the method used by Haffkine for his demonstration, Wright and Semple used heat to inactivate their cultures. Twenty-four-hour cultures of bacilli grown at "blood heat" (body temperature) were drawn into sterile glass pipettes. After the ends were sealed, the cultures were placed in a beaker of water heated to 60°C, a temperature sufficient to kill the organisms in five minutes. The vaccine was then tested for safety on eighteen (presumably) volunteers, sixteen of whom were medical officers "of the Army or Indian Medical Services, or upon surgeons on probation who were preparing to enter those services [as well as Wright and Semple themselves]." Individuals were identified only by initials. Presumably the initials A.E.W. and D.S. referred to Wright and Semple.[19]

The next challenge facing Wright and Semple was that of developing a safe yet accurate method of determining the efficacy of the vaccine they were testing. It would obviously have been unethical to intentionally expose human subjects to an agent which might potentially prove lethal if the vaccine was ineffective. And the epidemiological concept of prospective observations—observing over time whether any of the vaccinated men developed typhoid—was not yet widely applied in the study of infectious disease. Instead they chose to apply an observation previously demonstrated by Pfeiffer in the study of immunity to cholera, and Max von Gruber and Herbert Durham in preliminary work on diagnosis of typhoid fever (shortly developed in greater detail by Ferdnand Widal): the ability of immune serum to agglutinate bacteria:

> In order to appreciate the exact nature of the test ... and in order to form an exact estimate of its value, we have briefly to consider the basis upon which the method of serum diagnosis depends. Put briefly, that basis is to be found in the fact that whenever the micro-organisms which are casually associated with a specific fever are brought in contact with the serum or plasma of an animal or a patient who is undergoing, or who has undergone, an attack of the specific fever in question, the following succession of phenomena manifests itself: (a) The bacteria become agglutinated together, (b) the bacteria lose their mobility, (c) the clumps of agglutinated bacteria sink to the bottom, and the culture fluid, which was previously evenly turbid, becomes clarified; (d) the bacteria shrink up into the form of minute spherules, (e) lastly, the bacteria are definitely devitalized.
>
> For the purposes of serum diagnosis, it is not essential that this whole train of phenomena should come under observation. It suffices if any one of this series of phenomena comes distinctly under observation, provided always that we keep in view the fact that the subject matter of our

observations is no longer the actual bactericidal effect of the particular serum, but either its agglutinating, immobilizing, sedimenting, or spherulating effect. Provided we keep this in view, we shall be well advised if we, for purposes of serum diagnosis, select as the subject matter of our observations that particular effect which is most easily accessible to observation. Now as [Max von] Gruber and [Herbert] Durham were the first to show, the effect which is most accessible to observation is the agglomeration and the sedimentation of the bacteria. This effect can readily be appreciated by the unaided vision, even when, in accordance with the method which has been suggested by one of us ... minimal quantities of the serum and of the bacteria are mixed together in capillary sero-sedimentation tubes.

Having thus settled that the sedimentation of the bacteria is the phenomenon which will best serve as a criterion of a specific power of a serum, it will be obvious that we shall be able readily to determine in what measure the serum possesses this specific power if we make a series of successive dilutions of the serum, and determine how far the blood may be diluted without forfeiting its sedimenting powers.[20]

The principle was straightforward, and indeed would subsequently form the basis of the Widal test for diagnosis of typhoid. If immune serum was mixed with typhoid bacilli, substances—antibodies, as we now know—would combine with the bacilli causing them to agglutinate; if the clumps were sufficiently large they would sediment to the bottom of the tube. The level of the response in the subject would be a function of to what degree the serum could be diluted yet still be capable of providing visible agglutination: the greater the dilution, the stronger was the response in the host. Whether this would equate with immunity would still have to be determined.

The first inoculations with the "vaccine" were carried out between July and November 1896; most took place on November 20. As controls, serum samples were obtained just prior to vaccinations to observe a baseline of agglutination ability in the event that any of the subjects had previously been exposed to the bacillus; none of the tested samples demonstrated the ability to agglutinate. Results of the inoculations were promising. Serum from most of the subjects developed the ability to agglutinate typhoid bacilli, usually about five days after vaccination. Even samples diluted as much as 200-fold produced positive results.[21]

It was still uncertain, as the authors acknowledged, whether the ability to agglutinate (or sediment) also resulted in death of the microorganisms. Apparently it did not, as, when the authors tested agglutinated samples for survival, they found the bacilli were still viable. But even if the organisms were not killed in the glass tube (in vitro), could immune serum still exert such an "influence" on the microorganisms *in vivo*, that is, within the body? Here the inference was a possible yes. Test animals such as guinea pigs which had previously been immunized showed resistance to infection. Analogous experiments carried out on monkeys by Wright and David Bruce when studying Malta fever (brucellosis) had also shown protection against that disease when the animals had been immunized. Wright and Semple directly tested their idea on a subject designated "M.D." in their study. This person received three inoculations of the vaccine between July 31 and September 5, and his blood serum demonstrated significant agglutination ability. He was exposed to living, virulent typhoid bacilli on September 25 and, according to Wright, suffered no ill effects.[22]

Based on the aforementioned observations, Wright and Semple were able to declare, "We have the fact that, so far as we know, every convalescent from typhoid or Malta fever (and we may legitimately assume that such convalescents are, at any rate for a time, immune against reinfection with these specific fevers) shows a notable sedimentation reaction ... the only conclusion that can be reasonably deduced from this series of facts is the conclusion that the sedimenting power of the blood is a trustworthy criterion of the immunity of the patient who furnishes it. This conclusion cannot, however, be regarded as absolutely assured until we are in a position satisfactorily to account for the fact that the typhoid fever patients and Malta fever monkeys who succumb to these diseases show the specific sedimentation reaction in exactly the same way as the typhoid fever patients and Malta fever monkeys who recover from these diseases."[23]

So here was the conundrum. Even though volunteers vaccinated against typhoid produced serum capable of agglutinating the bacilli, similar properties were shown using serum from patients who succumbed to the disease. But Wright and Semple provided an explanation, some of which was prescient in its interpretation:

It would appear that every animal must be assumed to be working its way up to the acquirement of immunity from the very moment of infection to the time at which its struggle with the disease finally ceases. The sedimenting power of a patient, who afterwards succumbs to the disease, would thus appear to indicate only the degree of immunity which has been acquired at the particular moment at which blood was drawn off. And our experience of infective disease in general tells us that a degree of immunity which would, if already attained on the first day of the disease, amply suffice to ward off a fatal issue, will be of no avail if it is acquired later on in the course of the attack.... In the case of the typhoid or Malta fever patient, the sedimenting power of the blood may be acquired too late in the attack to save the patient's life.... We need no longer hesitate to accept, at least as a working hypothesis, the conclusion that the possession of a sedimenting power connotes also the possession of a certain measure of "bacteria proofness" against the bacteria in question.[24]

It was in statements following their explanation for the failure of agglutinating factors to always protect patients that Wright and Semple proved equally prescient. In attempting to explain a mechanism beyond simple killing power for the activity of these factors, the authors suggested the following: "We may reasonably surmise that this condition of bacteria proofness, inasmuch as it does not depend upon the presence of any absolutely bactericidal power in the blood, depends in large measure at least upon the fact that the typhoid bacilli which have been exposed to the poisonous influence of the blood fluids are likely to fall an easy prey to the phagocytes."[25] The vaccination procedure was not without its problems:

> About two or three hours after the injection a certain amount of local tenderness develops about the site of injection. This tenderness gradually increases in severity and extends upwards into the armpits and downwards into the groin. Corresponding with these subjective sensations a patch of congestion 2 to 3 inches in diameter develops round the site of the inoculation. Red lines of inflamed lymphatics can be distinctly traced, extending upwards into the armpits. The local tenderness is at its worst twelve hours after the injection.... Constitutional symptoms, consisting in some degree of faintness and collapse, begin to manifest themselves generally in two to three hours. In 4 out of 11 cases inoculated with these larger doses the faintness and nausea, resulting in one case in vomiting, were already well marked after three hours. In the other 7 cases these symptoms supervened somewhat later. Appetite was abolished. Only 3 out of the 11 cases were able to put in an appearance at dinner. A good deal of fever was developed in all cases, and sleep was a good deal disturbed.[26]

Fortunately none of the side effects proved serious in the long term; eight of the subjects were recovered by the following day, though the remainder required a period of several weeks for complete recovery.

A Role for Pfeiffer and Kolle

Did credit for development of the first practical vaccine against typhoid fever belong with Wright and Semple, or should equal credit be attributed to Richard Pfeiffer and Wilhelm Kolle? The former published their work in September 1896, while Pfeiffer and Kolle's report appeared two months later.[27] Furthermore, in the first paragraphs of the "Remarks on Vaccination," Wright and Semple stated, "Our first vaccinations against typhoid were undertaken in the months of July and August of last year

[1896]. These vaccinations were put on record by one of us in the *Lancet* on September 19, 1896, in a paper which dealt primarily with the question of serous hemorrhage. *A reprint of this paper was sent among others to Professor Pfeiffer.* "*Nearly two months after the date of this paper Professor Pfeiffer published, in conjunction with Dr. Kolle, a paper on Two Cases of Typhoid Vaccination* [italics added]. The method of inoculation which these authors have adopted, is exactly similar to the one that we had previously adopted. Like our own method, it was based upon the methods which have so successfully been employed by Mr. Haffkine in his anticholera inoculations."[28] In carrying out their own study, Pfeiffer and Kolle first confirmed the specificity of their typhoid cultures through agglutination reactions with immune serum and antityphoid serum prepared from a goat. After heat-killing the typhoid bacilli, inoculations were made in two individuals, named in their report as Eisenacher and Claudewitz. Other than minor reactions several hours later (a slight increase in temperature, chills, dizziness and tenderness at the site of injection), there were no significant side effects. When tested eleven days later, serum from each of the test subjects showed a significant increase in the ability to agglutinate typhoid bacilli, results analogous to those Wright and Semple had reported two months earlier.

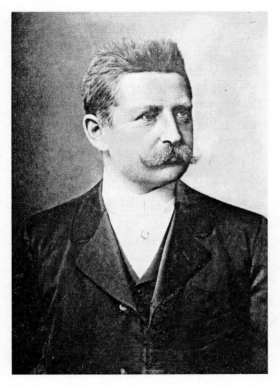

Richard Pfeiffer (1858–1945). Pfeiffer and his colleague, Wilhelm Kolle, tested a prototype typhoid vaccine at roughly the same time as Sir Almroth Wright did. It remains unclear whether Wright's work began as a modification of their procedure (courtesy Wellcome Library, London).

On the surface it appears Wright and Semple correctly deserve priority for developing the vaccination procedure. But in attempting to resolve the issue of priority one observation immediately stands out. In their concluding paragraph Pfeiffer and Kolle acknowledged the earlier work of others, notably Brieger, Wassermann and Fraenkel. Two researchers are not included in the short list: Wright and Semple. There are several possible explanations for what is admittedly negative evidence: (1) Pfeiffer and Kolle were unaware of their work, an unlikely supposition given the close interactions among researchers in the field; (2) Pfeiffer and Kolle chose to ignore the work, which is never cited in their report—again unlikely given the probable widespread knowledge of Wright's research on the subject; or (3) Pfeiffer and Kolle had carried out their inoculations of Eisenacher and Claudewitz prior to the summer and fall when Wright and Semple completed their work.

In their review of this same question of priority, Gröschel and Hornick provided an equally strong argument in favor of Pfeiffer and Kolle.[29] Some of their evidence rests on Wright's own words found in his typhoid fever treatise written seven years later. Under the heading "Question as to whether the inoculation of a typhoid culture which has been sterilized by exposure to temperatures of 60°C is capable of inducing in the organism the elaboration of the typhotropic substances which are required," Wright wrote as follows: "I may appropriately open the consideration of this question by pointing out the suggestion that preventive inoculations should be undertaken against typhoid fever upon the Pasteurian system [i.e., living attenuated bacilli]—a suggestion which was originally made to me by Mr. Haffkine—was, considering the risk which seemed to me to be involved in such a process, destined, so far as I was concerned, to remain indefinitely inoperative. The whole aspect of this suggestion was immediately changed as soon as I learned in the course of conversation with Professor R. Pfeiffer that

Wilhelm Kolle (1868–1935). Kolle and his colleague Richard Pfeiffer developed an early version of a typhoid vaccine similar to that produced by Sir Almroth Wright (courtesy National Library of Medicine).

he had in man obtained the specific agglutination-reaction to typhoid by the subcutaneous inoculation of a heated typhoid culture. This observation, since it pointed to the continued presence of effective vaccinating elements in the heated culture, immediately supplied the basis for the system of anti-typhoid inoculation which I have employed."[30] Wright thus acknowledged a contribution by Pfeiffer in the form of a suggested procedure for inactivation of live bacilli. But then in a footnote to his statement Wright seems to slightly backtrack: "It may be observed that Professor Pfeiffer also recognized that his observation with regard to the production of agglutinins by inoculation of sterilized cultures had opened the way to anti-typhoid inoculation. The results of two experimental anti-typhoid inoculations [i.e., Eisenacher and Claudewitz] were published by him in conjunction with Kolle (*Deutsche Medic. Wochenshft*, Nov. 12, 1896) shortly after the publication of my first two anti-typhoid inoculations (*Lancet*, September 19, 1896)."[31] As pointed out by Gröschel, the September 1896 publication by Wright in the *Lancet* dealt primarily with the use of calcium in alleviation of side effects (serous hemorrhage) following vaccination procedures; the inclusion of the test using a prototype vaccine on two army officers appears almost as an afterthought. Among other pieces of evidence included by Gröschel and Hornick in their review were statements attributed to Ernst Friedberger, a lecturer at Pfeiffer's Institute of Hygiene at the University of Königsberg. In 1907 in defense of the role played by Pfeiffer and Kolle, Friedberger disputed Wright's claim that it was Wright who first tested a vaccine. The arguments went back and forth, and in reality there is no defining element to resolve the issue of priority. It is best to accept the conclusion provided by Gröschel and Hornick: "It seems apparent that several groups were working on typhoid vaccine at the same time and the credit for using typhoid as a vaccine should be shared by the British [i.e., Wright] and the German [i.e., Pfeiffer and Kolle] workers."[32]

Explaining the Antibacterial Function of Serum

Wright and Semple were correct in their interpretation of the *in vivo* role played by the agglutinating factors, now known to be antibodies. It was several years later that Wright and Stewart Douglas, a captain in the Indian Medical Service with whom Wright became acquainted during his later work with the Indian Plague Commission (see below), were able to produce experimental support for Wright and Semple's original hypothesis that factors in immune serum contribute to phagocytosis.

By the turn of the century, even given the advances which had taken place in the nascent field of immunology, the actual function of body fluid itself in the antibacterial process remained uncertain. Paul Ehrlich and his colleagues had demonstrated the presence of a factor in immune serum which could lyse bacteria, a component initially called alexin but later termed complement. Elie Metchnikoff had demonstrated a role of white cells in the process of phagocytosis as well. But the relationship between the process of phagocytosis and agglutinating factors in immune system was still unresolved. It was in the context of this background that Wright and Douglas provided an explanation, coining a new immunological term in the process.

Their experimental procedure was straightforward. "White blood corpuscles" (phagocytes), bathed in either plasma or serum, were mixed with staphylococcal bacteria in sealed capillary tubes, and the average number of bacterial cells ingested by the phagocytes was measured. Wright and Douglas found that the level of phagocytosis when using unheated serum in which the cells were immersed was 10–15 times greater than when using heated serum. Their conclusion was "that the blood fluids modify the bacteria in a manner which renders them a ready prey to the phagocytes. We may speak of this as an 'opsonic' effect [opsono—I cater for; I prepare victuals for], and we may employ the term 'opsonins' to designate the elements in the blood fluids which produce this effect."[33] This was the first time the term "opsonin" was used to refer to substances in serum which enhance phagocytosis. But what actually were these substances? As we now understand, antibodies function in exactly that manner, coating the target and in turn binding to receptors on phagocytic cells. In effect, antibodies act as a bridge between the effector cell (phagocyte) and its target (in these examples, bacteria). The molecular mechanism was still unknown in the early 1900s but this was likely the role played by the agglutinating factors observed by Wright and Semple.

But the role of agglutinating factors—antibodies—was probably not the explanation for the results observed six years later by Wright and Douglas. First, the sources of the serum were finger pricks from the authors themselves; it was likely they were not dealing with antibodies in the serum against the staphylococci. The serum which was heated and which subsequently showed no enhancement of phagocytosis had been incubated for 10–15 minutes at 60–65°C, a treatment which might or might not have denatured antibody, but which certainly would have inactivated complement. Components of complement, or more properly components within the complement pathway, also act as opsonins. The conclusion must be that the opsonization observed by Wright and Douglas could be attributed to either antibodies, or, arguably more likely, proteins within the complement pathway. Regardless of which molecules served as opsonins, Wright and Douglas provided an accurate explanation for the role of immune serum in immunity.

Field Testing the Vaccine

In the concluding remarks of their description of their antityphoid vaccine, Wright and Semple included suggestions for proper testing of their product (in effect, proper field testing): "We venture to suggest that it would be expedient for every one who is likely to be frequently exposed to the risk of typhoid infection to undergo the vaccination. In particular this would appear to be expedient in the case of young soldiers going abroad to typhoid infected districts, to nurses who are in attendance upon typhoid patients, and, lastly, to persons who are living in any district which is being visited by an epidemic of typhoid."[34]

The first significant test of Wright's vaccine may have been during the Maidstone outbreak late in 1897. Between mid–August 1897 and January 1898, the town of Maidstone, Kent, suffered what was then the largest outbreak of typhoid fever in the country. Some 1,847 persons were reportedly infected, with 132 deaths.[35] The source of the epidemic, according to the local medical officer of health, appeared to have been the water supply from the reservoir at nearby Barming. The proximal cause may have been associated with a breakdown in sanitation testing:

> The town was supplied by the Maidstone Water Company, a private enterprise. The pumping station was at the bridge over the R, Medway. Water was obtained from several springs: at Tutsham and Ewell, west of the pumping station at Farleigh Bridge, and at Cossington and Boarley, north of Maidstone, at the foot of the North Downs. Before 1896 samples of the supply had been tested at monthly intervals but the Town Council, in the interests of economy, had reduced this to quarterly.... The last samples to be tested before the epidemic were in June. Later, a local newspaper commented that the epidemic was the penalty of such economy.
>
> Epidemiological investigations showed that there had been 1583 cases among customers supplied with water from the Farleigh area (Tutsham and Ewell), but only 29 and 69 respectively from the springs at Cossington and Boarley. There was also evidence of gross faecal contamination of the area around Tutsham spring. There were hop gardens nearby and accommodation for the hop-pickers was highly unsatisfactory and the sanitary facilities were non-existent. The hop-pickers defaecated anywhere.[36]

The obvious implication here is that the hop-pickers were responsible for the outbreak. However, it was also pointed out that the outbreak may have begun several days prior to their arrival, assuming the dates are accurate. Regardless of when it occurred, it is clear sanitation procedures left much to be desired.

Among the sites which obtained their water from the Barming reservoir was the Barming Lunatic Asylum (Kent County Lunatic Asylum). Prior to Wright's arrival, there had been 12 cases of typhoid among the 200 members of the staff. The vaccine was offered to 200 persons, with 84 accepting Wright's offer. None of the inoculated members developed typhoid, while among the 116 who were not vaccinated, 4 persons became ill.[37] While the total number of immunized individuals was not high, the efficacy of the vaccine did look promising.

A more efficacious opportunity to test the usefulness of Wright's vaccine presented itself late in 1898. Despite decreases in water-borne diseases such as dysentery among British troops stationed in India—the result of improved sanitation procedures—the incidence of typhoid continued to increase. In the period between 1889 and 1898, the incidence of the disease had increased from 1,093 reported cases in 1889 to 2,375 by 1898; deaths had increased from 283 to 657. In November 1898 Wright was appointed to the Indian Plague Commission, a commission of inquiry. Professor Thomas Fraser from Edinburgh University was appointed as president. The commission was sent to India with the purpose of investigating an outbreak of bubonic plague among the general population as well as that of typhoid among British troops. The investigation provided the opportunity to test his vaccine on a grander scale.[38]

It appeared almost as if those in charge of sanitation procedures for the army had learned little from the experience of the British army a generation earlier during the Crimean War. Open latrines were common, and in the absence of proper facilities men often urinated directly on the ground. Flies and other vermin had ready access to the untreated and open latrines and from there could easily contaminate food supplies. Once a soldier became infected it became nearly inevitable that the disease would be transmitted to others.

The initial report describing the efficacy of the vaccine covered the period roughly between Wright's arrival with the commission in late 1898 and the end of 1899.[39] The work carried out by Wright involved no shortage of challenges—not only technical problems such as preparation of the vaccine, but also the statistical analysis which followed. Compounding Wright's tasks was that even though the plague commission consisted of five scientists, apparently it was primarily Wright who took responsibility for producing the final report.[40]

Wright carried out all the preparations and inoculations himself—with the exception of the independent inoculation of the Royal Scots Corps stationed in Poona, which vaccinated an additional 172 troops—while also continuing his work with the plague commission. The route followed by the commission was that of a series of military stations, and it was at these that Wright inoculated army volunteers. The first challenge in this regard was producing sufficient vaccine:

> Owing to the fact that very little time was available before departure from England no sufficient supply of anti-typhoid vaccine could be prepared before starting. It was therefore necessary to manufacture vaccine *en route* during the intervals which occurred in the course of the sittings of the Plague Commission in Calcutta and Agra respectively. In these places the resources of local laboratories, presided over in the one case by Mr. Nield Cook [Medical College, Calcutta] and in the other case by Mr. Hankin [*sic*] [British bacteriologist Dr. Ernest Hanbury], were in the most generous manner placed at my disposal for the purpose of making the vaccine. The vaccine was standardized on guinea-pigs which were carried about from place to place for the purpose of keeping them continuously under observation. Inasmuch as the bottles of vaccine had to be opened up repeatedly for the purpose of drawing off the material, and inasmuch as it was not possible to carry about an incubator to verify the continued sterility of the vaccine, this last was re-sterilized at 60°C previously to undertaking each new series of inoculations.[41]

As discussed in greater depth by Dunnill, neither the government of India nor the British commander-in-chief, Sir William Lockhart (November 1898–March 1900), was consulted prior to implementation of the vaccination program.[42] Once the commander-in-chief and government of India became aware of what Wright was doing, the vaccination program was stopped. In spite of the abbreviated program, Wright reported that a total of 2,835 men were inoculated, with another 8,460 men serving as uninoculated "controls" for the purpose of statistical analysis of the results.[43] Wright conceded that the numbers available for statistical purposes were subject to a level of interpretation:

> The statistical material which is presented ... has been compiled from information furnished to me by officers of the Royal Army Medical Corps [established only in 1898] actually in charge of troops in the various stations. This information has been supplemented by reports received from the commanding officers of the various inoculated regiments.... This last task has not been freed from difficulty owing, among other things, to the fact that the various regiments are, in the hot season, broken up into detachments which are dispersed in the various hill stations.
> Taken as a whole the statistical material given herewith, though it cannot

from the nature of the case be assumed to be either complete or free from errors, would appear to show conclusively that a certain measure of protection was conferred by the inoculation of the quantities of dead typhoid culture which have been specified.... In appraising the amount of that protection from the data ... the following facts must not be lost sight of: 1. The inoculated men in the above units were, taken as a whole, in practically every case men who were much more likely to contract typhoid fever than the uninoculated men; for in practically every case the inoculated consisted to a large, and sometimes to a preponderating, extent of young men who had only recently come out to India, while the uninoculated consisted to a very great extent of older, more seasoned—in other words, of less susceptible—individuals.

2. It must be further borne in mind in connexion [*sic*] with certain of the statistics which have been given above that the inoculations were in certain cases undertaken in the actual presence of a typhoid fever epidemic.... In conformity with the fact that inoculations were done in these cases in the presence of typhoid fever it was only to be expected that some of the inoculated would prove to have been incubating typhoid fever at the time of the inoculation.[44]

So what were the actual results of the vaccination program carried out during these months as described by Wright? Of the 2,835 men vaccinated, 27 were diagnosed with typhoid (0.95 percent); of the 8,460 men not inoculated but observed for illness, 213 were diagnosed with the disease (2.5 percent).[45]

By the end of the century another series of events quickly provided an additional opportunity for Wright to test his vaccine, events which again involved the military. But this time the potential victims were beyond those of simply a colonial force. The Boer War (actually more accurately the second such war in twenty years in southern Africa) which began in October 1899, was in reality a continuation of the conflict which had begun nearly a century earlier in southern Africa between Afrikaans-speaking Dutch settlers and the British Empire. The actual history of the conflict—which ultimately resulted in a British victory by 1902—is complex and beyond the realm of this immediate topic. But as with most wars during that era, disease created a toll as large or greater than actual battlefield casualties. According to official British statistics, of the 556,653 men who served in the war, 57,684 contracted typhoid, an incidence of over 10 percent; there were 8,225 deaths from the disease. By comparison, 7,582 deaths were from battle wounds.[46] The Boers, on the other hand, were less affected by the disease, most likely because, unlike the British forces, which for much of the early period of the war remained in place, they were constantly on the move and consequently less affected by sanitation issues.

The question becomes whether typhoid inoculations were effective in limiting the extent of the disease, as extensive as it was. The siege of Ladysmith provided one opportunity to study the effectiveness of vaccination. During the early weeks of the war, Boer forces surrounded a British garrison in the town of Ladysmith consisting of some 12,500 troops. What became known as the Siege of Ladysmith lasted 118 days until the garrison were relieved at the end of the following February; among those in the garrison was a bacteriologist and colleague of Wright's, Dr. David Bruce, and his wife, Lady Bruce. In fact, Bruce had been placed in charge of the hospital where, according to a letter sent by his wife to her brother, at one point there were 1,000 patients admitted with typhoid. Bruce himself may have also become a victim.[47]

The results of vaccination, to use Wright's words, "would appear to be distinctly encouraging."[48] Of the 10,529 officers and men who did not receive the vaccination, 1,489 were subsequently diagnosed with typhoid, approximately 1 in 7.07. Among the 1,705 who received the inoculation, 35 were subsequently diagnosed with the disease: 1 in 48.7. A similar proportion was observed when calculating mortality from the disease. The risk of death among those vaccinated would appear to have been approximately one seventh that of the uninoculated, supporting Wright's contention for the efficacy of the vaccine.

The interval between inoculation and possible exposure to the typhoid agent is relevant: the greater the time interval, the more likely the men had developed a minimal level of immunity. In Wright's analysis it is unclear as to exactly when the inoculations had taken place. One can rule out vaccination during the actual siege, as Wright would not have been on the scene and supplies could not have been brought to the garrison anyway. Unfortunately, in the more complete description of the vaccination program provided by Wright is the time interval indicated.[49] The most likely possibility is that at least some of the inoculations had taken place while troops were onboard the transports, and others were inoculated once the army was being assembled. Wright included the possibility that the efficacy of the vaccine was even greater than the evidence from the statistics he provided, that the "role of typhoid fever among the inoculated" may have actually been fewer than the numbers suggested:

> The following points must be kept in view: 1. So far as is known the men who are set down as inoculated were with hardly an exception only once inoculated. It seems probable from the fact that only two cases among twice inoculated persons have as yet come to my knowledge that second inoculation confers a considerable additional protection [in effect, a booster shot,

in modern parlance]. 2. It is possible that certain of the officers who are set down as inoculated may have been inoculated with anti-typhoid serum and not with a vaccine consisting of a sterilized typhoid culture. [Wright suggests that some inoculations may have been that of serum instead of the actual vaccine.] Two or three instances have been reported to me where this error was committed in the case of officers proceeding to South Africa. In the statistics now in question the date and place of inoculation are in the case of five out of the nine officers attacked set down as unknown. 3. It is possible in the case of the men as distinguished from the officers that re-vaccination against smallpox, which, like anti-enteric inoculation, was in many cases carried out on board the transports may in certain instances have been confused with the latter inoculation. Instances of this confusion have already several times come to my knowledge [i.e., officers who received a smallpox vaccination might have mistaken this for the antityphoid inoculation in their reports]. 4. Lastly, it is possible that owing to the exigencies of military service or owing to other reasons the full prescribed dose of typhoid vaccine may not in all cases have been injected. Instances of the employment of the vaccine in fourfold reduced doses have come to my knowledge....

In view of the above points, regarding which there is not at present any information available, it is at present impossible to determine precisely to what extent the inoculated were protected by inoculation. But the results set forth ... would appear to be distinctly encouraging, inasmuch as they show that the proportion, on the one hand, of attacks, and on the other hand of deaths, from typhoid fever was seven times smaller in the inoculated than in the uninoculated. And it may be borne in mind that if the number (no doubt a considerable one) of men who had previously suffered from typhoid fever had been subtracted from the number of the uninoculated, as quite legitimately have been done, the statistics would have borne an even more favorable aspect.[50]

Wright's interpretation of the efficacy of his vaccine was certainly not universally accepted. Partly as the result of vaccine which was often variable in strength—dilution was alluded to in Wright's report above—and the fact that some soldiers received an additional booster inoculation, some people felt the results were as much due to chance as they were to the efficacy of the vaccine. In addition, the vaccine sometimes produced unpleasant side effects, in some cases due either to lack of sterility or as the result of an overdose, and as a consequence many soldiers refused to be inoculated. In at least one instance, the response to the vaccine was more drastic: "A supply of the vaccine was dispatched with the troops bound for the Boer War, though without a clear official blessing. Some of it was dumped overboard in Southampton Water, lest it cause disease, and was returned to Wright by the coastguards."[51]

Despite the controversies which the use of Wright's vaccine had generated, the reality was, to use a cliché, that one can't argue with success. Once preparation of the vaccine had been standardized (one immediate change was to inactivate at a temperature of 53°C rather than 60°C) it became clear that it was effective, perhaps at not completely eliminating typhoid fever, but in significantly reducing the incidence of the disease. The particular strain of bacillus, known as the Rawlings strain, which would serve as the prototype vaccine, was also standardized. The organism had been isolated from a fatal case of the illness and was found to produce fewer unpleasant side effects when used as a vaccine.

There were several immediate tests which were applied elsewhere. The German Colonial Army (the Schutztruppe) instituted a vaccination campaign during their suppression of the Herero peoples of Southwest Africa (Namibia) in the 1904–1907 war. Reportedly, the incidence of typhoid among the inoculated troops was less than 50 percent of that in the uninoculated men.[52] Ironically, the German army failed to implement the vaccine during the first months of the Great War, which began in the following decade, resulting in an outbreak of the disease before mandatory vaccination was instituted.

As described in a subsequent chapter, typhoid fever took a heavy toll in 1898 among United States troops training in the southeastern United States prior to embarkation during the Spanish-American War. The Typhoid Commission, which investigated the outbreak, took note of the abysmal sanitary practices that had resulted in the epidemic, which according to government figures affected approximately 21,000 troops, with 2,200 deaths. The voluntary use of the vaccine by the army was instituted in 1909, with mandatory vaccination introduced in 1911. The vaccine and introduction of proper sanitary practices resulted in there being no significant typhoid morbidity among U.S. troops during World War I.

Sir Almroth Edward Wright (1861–1947)

Almroth Edward Wright was born August 10, 1861, in Middleton Tyas, the second of five sons to the Reverend Charles Wright, then curate of the parish, and Ebba Almroth, whose late father had served both as director of the Swedish Royal Mint and as professor of chemistry at the Royal Military School at Marieburg (Sweden). Wright spent much of his early life moving from place to place, first as a result of his father's vocation and then as a student, fifteen years of which were spent in Ireland developing a profession. Wright's grammar training was at the Belfast Academical Institution, which was followed in 1878 by enrollment in Trinity College in Dublin. Graduating four years later with first-class honors in modern literature and a gold medal while also developing an interest in medicine, it was at Trinity that Wright's skepticism of much of "modern" medical practice began to mature.

Wright's interest in learning experimental medicine led him to Leipzig, where, aided by a traveling scholarship, he had the opportunity to briefly work with fellow Englishman Leonard Wooldridge in the study of blood coagulation, a collaboration which would resume several years later. His sojourn in Germany also provided an opportunity to observe some of the "giants" in the field of physiology, including Carl Ludwig and Julius Connheim. Returning to England, in part as a result of a shortage of funds, Wright passed an examination for civil service which resulted in a paid appointment in 1885 to a clerkship in law for the Admiralty. In his spare time Wright continued his interest in medicine as an (unpaid) assistant for Wooldridge, continuing to study blood coagulation, and Victor Horsley, with whom he studied both blood coagulation and the function of the thyroid gland at the Brown Animal Sanctuary Institution in Wandsworth. The Brown Sanctuary was a research institution outside of London established through the will of Thomas Brown for ostensibly "investigating, studying, and without charge beyond immediate expenses, endeavoring to cure maladies, distempers and injuries any quadrupeds or birds useful to man may be subject to."[53] The position provided an opportunity for Wright to learn firsthand procedures which would prove useful in his later career. Exhibiting the independent streak for which he would be well known, a perceived lack of diligence at the Admiralty might have cost Wright his position there had he not two years later accepted an offer by Dr. Charles Roy, chair of the department, of a demonstratorship in pathology at Cambridge.[54]

During these early years as a young man developing expertise in his profession, without the responsibility yet of a family, Wright spent much of his time traveling between various research laboratories, and not always of his own volition. He later admitted, "I could never say a modest thing in all my life ... [and] the respectability and conventional ways of Cambridge were anathema."[55] During his two years at Cambridge he obtained a Grocer's Company scholarship which allowed him to travel to Germany, where he received further experience in the fields of anatomy and physiology as well as in physiological chemistry. In 1889 Wright accepted an appointment to a demonstratorship in physiology in Sydney, Australia. But there had occurred a significant change in his personal life by then: in 1889 he married Jane Georgina Wilson. The two sailed for Australia late that year. There Wright continued to carry out studies on blood coagulation, later continued in parallel with analogous studies with milk (see above) as well as acidosis as a consequence of diabetes. But once again dissatisfaction with his work led Wright to decide another move was necessary, and early in 1891 he returned to England with his growing family, this time for a position at the Royal College of Physicians and Surgeons, where he would study the chemistry of fibrinogen.

Wright's appointment was fortuitous. The superintendent was the pathologist German Sims Woodhead, later a president of the Royal Medical Society, the author of the textbook *Practical Pathology* (1883), and a man with military connections. When Woodhead was asked to recommend a pathologist for the army's Royal Victoria Hospital at Netley it was Wright's name he put forward.[56]

Wright became professor of pathology at Netley in 1892, at which time he became a member of a group known as Surgeons on Probation, largely composed of physicians in training from either

Sir Almroth Wright (1861–1947). Wright is generally credited with development of the first effective vaccine against typhoid fever, though an argument may be made that Pfeiffer and Kolle deserve priority. Nevertheless, Wright's field studies with the British forces demonstrated its usefulness in providing protection against the disease (courtesy Wellcome Library, London).

the Indian Medical Service or from the research department of the government of India. Among those with future prominence were David Semple, who, as related earlier, was an important colleague of Wright's in development of the typhoid vaccine, and (Sir) William Leishman, future director-general of Army Medical Services who is also known for the isolation and identification of the etiological agent of kala azar, a protozoan named *Leishmania*.[57]

Wright's work in the development of the typhoid vaccine as well as his participation in the plague commission, beginning in 1898, which allowed him to test his vaccine on a larger scale, are related above. Despite some of the controversy over the use and efficacy of his vaccine, the British military adopted the procedure, which proved particularly important during the Great War, which began in 1914. The numbers tell the story when comparing the incidence of the disease during the Boer War with that between 1914 and 1918.[58] Better sanitation procedures certainly played a part, though conditions in the trenches were far from ideal in that respect. It appears clear that Wright's vaccine helped significantly reduce the incidence of typhoid, as can be seen in the table below.

	Annual Incidence/1000	Annual Death Rate/1000	Total Cases	Total Deaths	Mean Strength
Boer War (1899–1902)	105.00	14.6	57,684	9,022	208,226
The Great War (1914–1918)	2.35	0.139	20,139	1,191	ca. 2,000,000

In 1906 Wright was knighted for his contributions. By then he had left Netley, becoming professor of pathology at St. Mary's Hospital, London, in 1902, where he would serve as director until he retired some 45 years later. Among the colleagues associated with him were Stewart Douglas, whose work with Wright established the role of opsonins in immune function (previously discussed), as well as Alexander Fleming, credited with discovery of the antibacterial substances lysozyme and penicillin in the years after the war.

As important a figure as Wright was, he was not without controversy. His views on the role of women in science and public life in general were an extreme reflection of the general 19th century attitude (see *The Unexpurgated Case Against Woman Suffrage*, 1913). He was largely skeptical about the use of antibiotics in treating disease, believing that pathogens would quickly become resistant; ironically, on that front, he has increasingly been proven correct. Instead, he was a strong advocate of preventive medicine, of which the development of vaccines was an example. Almost until his death at the age of eighty-six Wright continued his research, which included studying methods to grow the tuberculosis bacillus as well as investigating the process of phagocytosis.

Typhoid Vaccines in the Postwar Era

Several modifications of the vaccines in use by the military took place in the years following the end of World War II. The heat-phenol inactivated cultures remained the standard for some time in the American army, while an alcohol-inactivated version was used by the British military. At the same time, studies carried out at the Walter Reed Army Medical School showed that an acetone-killed and dried (AKD) vaccine might be more effective.[59] The primary problems with each of these vaccines were the side effects which often followed the procedure: localized inflammation at the site of injection as well as common febrile reactions. In addition, the inactivated version required two injections. Even this procedure conferred immunity for only a short period of time. The next generation of vaccines, developed during the 1980s and 1990s, was able to circumvent some of these complications.

The first of these, a live attenuated strain of *Salmonella typhi*, termed Ty21a, was first licensed in Europe in 1983 and in the United States in 1989. The mutated parent strain, developed in 1975, lacks an enzyme, uridine diphosphate-galactose-4-epimerase. As a result, it is unable to metabolize the sugar galactose properly. Derivatives of galactose form toxic byproducts which lyse the cells.[60] The original strain was isolated on the basis of the inability to metabolize the sugar. Subsequent chemically induced mutations have inactivated additional genes, including the gene encoding what is known as the Vi (virulence) antigen, a polysaccharide which normally protects the bacterium from the host's immune system (see below). While the organism is unable to produce the disease, it is sufficiently immunogenic to induce protective immunity. A major advantage of this vaccine is that it can be taken orally, which is particularly helpful when immunizing children. However, maximum protection still requires a series of three doses.

The alternative classes of modern typhoid vaccines consist of modified forms of the Vi antigen. The name applied to the polysaccharide reflected its importance in the pathogenicity of *Salmonella*. The discovery of the Vi antigen by Arthur Felix and Margaret Pitt from the Lister Institute in London during the 1930s represented a significant advance in the understanding of the immune response to a bacterial infection.[61]

Bacteria such as *Salmonella typhi*, then referred to by the genus and species name of *Bacillus typhosus*, were known to express two significant antigens which trigger an immune response. The O polysaccharide represents the sugars on the surface of the cell, while the H antigen represents the proteins of the flagella. The immune response to the O antigen is the more important factor in protecting the infected host. Felix and Pitt observed that the level of virulence associated with the bacterium is a function of the ability of the host to respond to infection. Strains which were agglutinated by antibody against the O antigen were largely avirulent, while strains in which antibody against the O antigen did not cause agglutination were highly virulent. This was the result even though the O polysaccharide moiety of each variant was identical. Felix and Pitt's conclusion was that "the mere presence of … O antigen does not of itself determine high virulence, and that some unknown factor is required to render this antigen resistant to the action of the O antibody."[62]

For the experiments in which Felix and Pitt identified the protective factor, two highly virulent strains and two avirulent strains were heat killed and inoculated into mice. Only the inactivated highly virulent strains induced protective antibody against living bacteria, indicating the factor responsible for protecting the bacteria from the host immune system was a separate antigen from that of either O or H and was heat resistant. The newly recognized factor was dubbed the Vi (for virulence) antigen, and was associated with capsular material produced by the bacterium. Further experiments by Felix and Pitt confirmed that the Vi antigen was unique and not part of the O polysaccharide. In the absence of the virulence antigen, antibody directed against the O polysaccharide is capable of agglutinating those strains, and is protective in the host—explaining why those strains are avirulent. The presence of the Vi antigen serves to protect the bacteria from antibody against the O polysaccharide, explaining the virulence of those strains. The logical question which followed was whether a vaccine composed of the Vi antigen itself would be effective against typhoid fever.

An extensive pilot study followed by a clinical trial of the effectiveness of a Vi vaccine was carried out during the mid–1980s. In the initial pilot study, 274 Nepalese received a vaccine composed of purified Vi capsular material. No significant side effects were observed, and 75 percent of the participants were found to produce protective levels of antibody. The follow-up clinical trial involved nearly 7,000 persons, with similar results. Most participants (~75 percent) produced protective levels of antibody, a level which was disappointing to the physicians, but still it was nevertheless sufficient for demonstrating the efficacy of the vaccine.[63] The typhoid Vi polysaccharide vaccine was licensed in the United States in 1994.

One of the reasons the vaccine was less effective than hoped was the nature of the molecule. Polysaccharides such as the Vi antigen often do not invoke a strong immune response, unlike the situation with protein antigens. In the past, conjugate vaccines composed of polysaccharide chemically attached to a protein carrier had proven more effective as a vaccine,[64] and a similar procedure was subsequently carried out with the Vi antigen attached to a protein carrier. A conjugate vaccine in which the Vi polysaccharide was linked to a protein similar to one produced by the bacterium *Pseudomonas aeruginosa* was found to be more effective than the Vi antigen by itself.[65] The current conjugate vaccine (2014) is similar to that previously tested, and consists of the Vi antigen coupled to tetanus toxoid. The vaccine is used only in areas of the world, such as Southeast Asia, where typhoid fever is endemic.

The evolution of typhoid vaccine development largely took place within a century, beginning with the work of Wright and Pfeiffer (it would be unfair to claim priority for either) in the late 19th century and culminating with the conjugate vaccines of the late 20th century. The procedures mimic those of the field of bacteriology in general, starting with heat inactivation of the typhoid bacilli and ending with techniques of molecular biology using isolated components of the organism. In the United States the time period of development was even shorter and would be within the lifetime of many individuals. The first vaccine for the general public was licensed in 1914, and the first Vi polysaccharide vaccine was licensed 80 years later. This was followed after a few years by the conjugate version.

11

Typhoid in the American Army

The history of typhoid vaccination in the United States Army began in May 1904 when James Carroll, then a First Lieutenant and Director of Laboratories at the Army Medical School, proposed the vaccination of soldiers by the oral administration of dead typhoid bacilli.—Dr. Edward Vedder, Professor of Pathology and Preventive Medicine, George Washington University (1935). (December 9, 1935: "Publication denied for reasons of public policy.")[1]

We have seen in the previous chapter how the vaccine developed by Wright was instrumental in controlling the outbreak of typhoid fever among men in the British army by the time of the Boer War. What of the American army? Of course the situations had their differences. British forces were involved primarily in maintaining a colonial empire; the phrase "the sun never sets on the British empire" had an element of truth at its core. Though perhaps not as frequently as in earlier centuries, British forces were involved in wars in far-flung areas during the nineteenth century. India and the Crimea are two prime examples. The United States had no significant colonial ambitions until long after the Civil War, and until the incursion into Cuba during the Spanish-American War in 1898 it was never involved in foreign entanglements. Nevertheless, any time that substantial numbers of soldiers were housed in situations in which sanitary precautions were ignored, the threat of disease was real.

Statistics on the incidence of typhoid among military personnel which cover the period between the Revolutionary War and the beginning of the Civil War are limited. The importance of the disease and its effects on military campaigns throughout history is well known, and there is certainly no reason to think American forces were spared during this period. This would be particularly true during those periods in which the army was in camp for an extended length of time. During the winter of 1777–1778, when Washington's army of some 11–12,000 men was at Valley Forge, over 2,000 soldiers died from exposure or diseases like dysentery and typhoid fever.

Anecdotal descriptions of actual illnesses such as smallpox and diarrheal diseases including the aforementioned dysentery and typhoid are well known. During the American Revolution, the army attempted to mitigate the impact of smallpox among the troops through variolation, the scarifying of skin using scabs of dried pocks obtained from persons recovering from mild cases. However, medical authorities did not keep track of smallpox or other common diseases until April 1818. That year, Dr. Joseph Lovell was appointed as the first surgeon general of the United States Army following the reorganization of the army staff, and the Medical Department was recognized as a staff department of that branch of service.[2] Even with the establishment of the medical department, numbers remained crude estimates; incidence rates for typhoid between 1820 and 1861 appear to have ranged between 2 and 10 per 1000 per annum. Estimates for the Civil War are likewise inexact and apply primarily to the Union armies. Somewhere over 2,000,000 men served the North during the war. An estimated 80,000 admissions for typhoid were recorded by the medical department, a number which undoubtedly was an underestimate. This would produce a morbidity rate upwards of 5 percent, and probably greater, given the quality of sanitation at the time. With the case fatality rate for the disease ranging between 5–10 percent, and extrapolating to a more realistic morbidity rate, it is likely a minimum of 25,000 soldiers died as a result of typhoid infection.[3] Though statistics for illness in the armies of the Confederacy are not available, it is likely that the incidence of the disease was comparable. Other diarrheal diseases were equally common; by the last year of the war the incidence of bowel disease as a whole among Union soldiers was 995 per 1000 men. The reason was obvious—contamination of water supplies with sewage from latrines. One graphic description of a Union camp reported "the camp sink [latrine] is located between the tents and the river. It is covered with fresh earth twice a week....The men, however, generally make use of the ground in the vicinity."[4]

The situation was no better in the cities, particularly in the early years of the war. In Washington, D.C., for example, "sanitary conditions were nightmarish. The Washington Canal, running through the middle of the city, became an open toilet, a receptacle for all the city's sewage—human, equine, and otherwise. It all found its way to the Potomac and, according to a government report, 'spread out in thinner proportions over several hundred acres of tidal flats immediately in front of the city, the surface of which is exposed to the action of the sun at intervals during the day, and the miasma from which contaminates every breath of air which passes.' The stench was everywhere."[5]

Record keeping by the time of the Spanish-American War was more systematic. Hence the statistics for determining the incidence of typhoid fever were more accurate. Typhoid was not the only disease the troops encountered during the Cuban campaign (mosquito-borne diseases such as yellow fever produced a casualty rate greater than Spanish bullets), but given the medical knowledge available by 1898, including that of the etiological agent of typhoid and its means of spread, the high incidence of the disease was that much more inexcusable. Only 243 troops died directly or indirectly as battle casualties; nearly 2,200 men died from typhoid fever. One of every five men in the army developed typhoid.[6]

The vast majority of typhoid infections among the troops occurred not while they were in combat in Cuba but while still in training camps located in the southeastern United States. Most of those cases were clustered in the summer and early fall of 1898. As a result of the widespread nature of the illness, the Typhoid Fever Board, consisting of Majors Walter Reed, Edward Shakespeare and Victor Vaughan, was established to investigate the underlying causes of the outbreak. These three physicians spent much of the late summer and early fall, from August 20 to September 30, traveling through seven volunteer army training camps to investigate sanitary procedures. The board produced a scathing report, which was published in 1904. Both Reed and Shakespeare were dead by then, the former from a ruptured appendix, the latter from heart disease, and it was Vaughan who wrote much of the final report. That report focused on two primary topics: confusion in the diagnosis of typhoid fever, and the abysmal sanitation procedures followed by medical personnel in the camps.

The first camp inspected by Reed, Shakespeare and Vaughan was Camp Alger in Dunn Loring, Virginia, located west of Arlington in the northeastern portion of the state. The members of the commission arrived during the last weeks of August and remained at the site for six days. The first day was spent, in part, simply locating a microscope and in finding assistants who could help properly diagnose the disease. As described previously in this history, cases of typhoid fever in the past had been often misdiagnosed as malaria (typhomalaria). While the diseases themselves were distinctly different—diagnosis of malaria would be predicated on identification of the malarial parasite, while typhoid could be determined through a positive Widal test—few of the medical personnel on hand could accurately differentiate the illnesses. Once qualified assistants were brought on board, among whom were Drs. William Gray and James Carroll from the Army Medical Branch, the confusion was eliminated. Nearly all cases reported as typhomalaria were actually typhoid fever.[7]

Though this solved the problem of identification at Camp Alger, medical officers at other camps continued to diagnose patients incorrectly. Rather than simply argue the cases with these physicians, Reed, Shakespeare and Vaughan decided to carry out what in modern parlance would be defined as a blinded study. When they arrived at Camp Cuba Libre in Jacksonville, Florida, they consulted with the commanding officer, Fitzhugh Lee (son of the late Confederate general Robert E. Lee), requesting that medical personnel at the camp select fifty cases of "typhomalaria" and send them to Fort Myer near Washington, D.C., to have the patients examined by Dr. Carroll. Carroll correctly diagnosed the illnesses as typhoid fever. Another one hundred and fifty men ill with "typhomalaria" were sent to other hospitals for examination; all confirmed the diagnosis of typhoid fever.[8]

The investigation by the Typhoid Board at Camp Cuba Libre also produced an explanation for the sudden appearance of the disease. By 1898 it was known that typhoid is usually spread through fecal contamination of the food or water supply. The initial assumption was that the water source for both the camp and the city, a series of four artesian wells, had somehow been polluted with human waste. However, the wells ranged in depth from six hundred feet to greater than one thousand feet, far too deep for fecal contamination from the soldiers' latrines to occur.[9] In addition, though the populations of Jacksonville and the camp were approximately equal—some 30,000 persons in each—the outbreak of typhoid was confined almost entirely among the soldiers.

The explanation was quickly obvious: the process by which fecal waste was removed from the camp. Disposal of the waste, by now often contaminated with bacteria which included the typhoid agent, was accomplished through a method called the tub system to clean the latrines. Waste was collected in old whiskey barrels, the contents of which were then dumped into larger barrels that were carried on wagons along bumpy roads. Both urine and fecal waste were collected in the mixture, and barrels were often filled to overflowing. Vaughan later described the process in a graphic manner: "The disposal of fecal matter from the sinks was by hauling in tubs, filled to overflowing and constantly slopping and spilling along this (shell) road within 20 feet of our tents, and generally at mealtime. It was impossible to keep the dust out of our food, and the passing of these filthy and vile smelling wagons while the men were eating was almost in itself cause enough for sickness, even had infectious germs been absent from the loathsome loads."[10] The members of the board recommended a solution which was quickly implemented. The tub system as a means of transporting fecal material was stopped, and latrines were routinely disinfected with lime. Once these changes were made, the epidemic of typhoid ended.

Similar procedures were carried out in other camps which had been subjected to outbreaks of typhoid. Camp George Thomas at Chickamauga Park, the site of one of the bloodiest battles of the Civil War, held as many as 60,000 men. Chickamauga Creek provided drainage for the camp, the troops of which produced some 9.4 tons of feces and 21,000 gallons of urine on a daily basis. Military orders covering proper sanitation procedures had been issued as early as the previous April by the surgeon general, George Sternberg. Camps were to be set up on high ground to allow for proper drainage, with each company to be in charge of constructing their own latrines. Latrines were to be treated a minimum of three times each day with either lime or ash and then covered. Water was to be boiled prior to use, obviously for both coffee and tea, but the order also applied to drinking water.

As has been the case with soldiers throughout history spending much of their spare time waiting for orders, instructions were increasingly ignored. Latrines often were simply shallow pits, untreated and uncovered. In some cases they were placed uphill from soldiers' tents. And even those latrines dug on the lower portions of hills became flooded during the rains that began in summer. The orders for boiling of drinking water were often disregarded. Arguably, the epitome of ignorance with respect to sanitary precautions was exhibited by members of one company: "A spring adjacent to the outpost near the Chickamauga Creek was flooded during the storms, leaving behind a coating of slime after the creek subsided. Acting upon the suggestion that germs floated, 'they plunged a canteen to the bottom of the spring, with the opening stopped by the thumb against the entrance of bacteria. When the canteen was on the bottom, the thumb was removed until the canteen was filled, the opening was then plugged with the thumb, and the supply brought to the surface.' Every person who drank from the spring came down with typhoid shortly afterward."[11]

An abstract of the report produced by the Typhoid Board was ready by 1900. The original plan was that Vaughan would provide analysis of the typhoid outbreak, while Reed and Shakespeare would produce the final copy. However, in mid–1900 Shakespeare died as a result of a sudden heart attack, leaving it to Reed and Vaughan to produce the final report. After

Reed himself died in 1902, Vaughan completed the report, which consisted of two volumes, in 1904.[12] The final report included fifty-seven determinations and recommendations. The sanitary procedures, or lack thereof, received particular attention. Vaughan had estimated that with typhoid as widespread as it was throughout the country it was inevitable that some new recruits would enter the camp while carrying the disease. In an average regiment consisting of 1,300 men, it was probable that one or several already were ill with the disease. The problem lay with the question of how one should properly eliminate the fecal excretions, over 9 tons each day, produced by 1,300 men. The Typhoid Board laid the blame for improper disposal on inexperienced medical officers who, in attempts to curry favor with the troops,

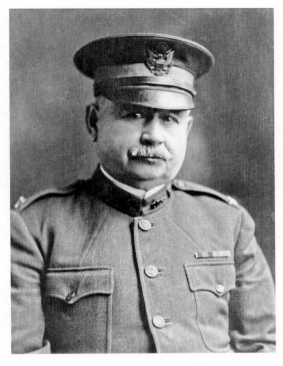

Victor Vaughan (1851–1929). Long-time chair of the medical school at the University of Michigan, Vaughan has been credited with modernizing the program. As a member of the Typhoid Commission in 1898, he helped determine the source of typhoid outbreaks among American troops (courtesy National Library of Medicine).

were lax in enforcement of sanitary procedures. In the future, human waste was to be collected in troughs containing milk of lime. The troughs would be cleaned on a daily basis.

Most of the board's (Vaughan's) recommendations were carried out. The results were observed after the United States entered World War I. The combination of proper sanitation as well as implementation of a new trivalent vaccine (see below) significantly reduced the incidence of typhoid fever; among the four million American troops serving in that war, only 1,529 were admitted to military hospitals with typhoid, fewer cases than had been found in some camps in 1898.[13] But even the implementation of the most basic sanitary precautions would take some time. The peacetime army of 1904 still reported an incidence of 5.14 typhoid cases per 1,000 per year, primarily among new recruits. Perhaps one explanation could be found in the surgeon general's report for 1905: "The issue of toilet paper is now authorized where posts have sewer connections."[14]

As recounted earlier, the first effective typhoid vaccine had been developed in the 1890s by either Sir Almroth Wright or Richard Pfeiffer, or simultaneously by each, using a heat-killed culture of typhoid bacilli. In 1904 a similar process was used by American officers in an attempt to duplicate the Wright and Pfeiffer results by preparing their own heat-killed culture. A description of the vaccine trial, the first to show that this particular trial had even taken place, was finally presented in some detail by Colonel William Tigertt in a 1959 publication in the journal *Military Medicine*.[15]

After obtaining permission for the test from the surgeon general of the army, Robert Maitland O'Reilly, Major James Carroll, Drs. Edward Vedder and Harry Lorenzo Gilchrist prepared the vaccine by heating a culture of typhoid bacilli at 56°C for one hour. Carroll had already risen to prominence as a result of his work several years earlier with Walter Reed in determining the role of the mosquito in transmission of yellow fever. At that time Carroll had been a member of the Board for the Investigation of Yellow Fever, serving as the initial "volunteer victim" to be bitten by the mosquito suspected of carrying the etiological agent. He was fortunate to survive the illness, which is thought to have contributed to his eventual death in 1907. Vedder was a graduate of the Army Medical School (1904) and would serve as Carroll's assistant. He would later become well known as a result of his work in the Philippines some years later when he proved that the illness beri-beri was associated with a nutritional deficiency rather than an infectious agent. He was appointed commandant of the Army Medical School in 1930. Gilchrist, by then a colonel, would head the American Typhus Relief Expedition to Poland in 1919. The following year he would be appointed to the position of chief medical officer of the Chemical Warfare Service. By 1929 he would head the medical branch of the army's chemical warfare service. The vaccine, prepared by heating the Dorset strain of *Bacillus typhosus* for one hour at 56°C, was to be taken orally by Carroll, Vedder, Gilchrist and ten volunteers[16]:

> The men were instructed to report at 2:00 p.m. on July 12, 1904. On the morning of the above date, the First Sergeant [Howe] reported to Lieutenant Gilchrist that the men who had volunteered to participate in the test had requested to be relieved. It appeared they had a presentiment that something was going to happen. They were instructed to report to the

Dispensary at the appointed place, day and hour and then if they wished to be excused, they could do so at the time.

In view of the misapprehension on the part of the men concerning this experiment, after they were assembled Lieutenant Carroll explained to them the value of the work in which they had volunteered to participate, and what the experiment, if successful, would mean not only to the Army but to the world at large. At the same time he said that although every known precaution was taken in the preparation of the vaccine, and tests on animals had shown it to be harmless, he could give no assurance that there would not be some reactions, but it was his opinion that they would not be serious.

In order to encourage the men [see *n* 14] to carry out this experiment Lieutenants Gilchrist and Vedder first took doses of the vaccine larger than those prescribed. Following this, the men lined up and each took 30 c.c. of the typhoid vaccine…. The men were instructed to report back in ten days for the second dose.[17]

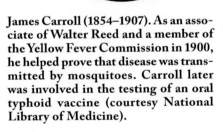

James Carroll (1854–1907). As an associate of Walter Reed and a member of the Yellow Fever Commission in 1900, he helped prove that disease was transmitted by mosquitoes. Carroll later was involved in the testing of an oral typhoid vaccine (courtesy National Library of Medicine).

The results when using the "vaccine" were considerably less than successful, as most of the men developed "typical" typhoid or a febrile illness which may very well have been typhoid. Carroll had been infected with typhoid some years earlier and, likely being already immune, showed no evidence of illness.[18] Neither Private Lumley nor Private Epps became ill. The other volunteers were not all as fortunate. By the beginning of August both Vedder and Gilchrist had developed fevers approaching 104°F, with rose spots appearing on their backs and abdomens, and they were hospitalized until the end of the month. Vedder in particular was diagnosed with "severe" typhoid fever. Sergeant Howe was the "least" ill among those with symptoms; the company clerk, Howe reportedly felt ill but exhibited a temperature only slightly above normal. The remaining men suffered a range of symptoms. Blood cultures for detection of either serum antibody or typhoid bacilli were carried out on only some of the men. But the exposure to the vaccine, the incubation period typical of typhoid, and of course the symptoms all support the claim that the men did indeed develop typhoid fever.[19]

The obvious question was how the men came to be exposed when the vaccine contained allegedly dead bacteria. When samples of the vaccine were plated on nutrient media, two or three colonies developed, indicating that live bacilli were also present in the vaccine despite the process of heat inactivation. It was also clear that even though the cultures had been maintained in the laboratory for six years, they had lost none of their virulence. When the inactivation process was repeated, it was found that, while the temperature of the cultivating medium

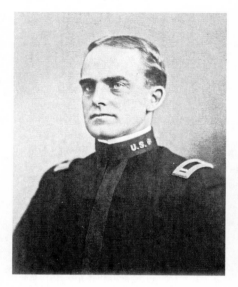

Harry Lorenzo Gilchrist (1879–1943). As an army physician, Gilchrist helped produce the typhoid vaccine subsequently tested on soldiers in 1904. The vaccine trial proved largely unsuccessful, as the vaccine had been improperly purified (courtesy National Library of Medicine).

reached 56°C on the outer portions of the (liter) flask, the inner portions may have had a temperature several degrees cooler, resulting in an incomplete inactivation. As noted in the quote which began this chapter, Vedder's attempt to describe this initial test was subjected to censorship for reasons which remain obscure. Despite this, Tigertt noted several conclusions which could be made, and later applied, from the vaccine trial: "(1) The organisms (Dorsett strain of typhoid bacilli) had been on artificial culture for six years; (2) The infecting dose for man was small and produced typical disease in at least 7 of 12 presumed susceptibles; and (3) The simultaneous ingestion of a large number of killed organisms along with the few viable cells had no appreciable salutary influence on the disease picture."[20]

Four years later the medical branch of the army was ready to try again. In 1908 Major Frederick Russell was sent to England to visit with Wright in order to determine the optimal method of vaccine preparation as well as the proper dose to utilize. Among the changes implemented by Russell was that of heating smaller doses of the typhoid bacillus to achieve more uniform inactivation. As described by Russell several years later (1913), once the vaccine had been implemented within the army, the efficacy and safety of the Rawlings strain of the vaccine originally used by the British met the required standards:

In [March] 1909 we began the treatment after submitting the matter to a board of officers, as we desired the support of the medical profession of the country. It was a subject of the greatest importance. We could not afford another experience like that of the Spanish-American War.

But volunteers for the experiments were not readily obtained. The vaccine was first tried on the laboratory staff. Then the medical officers in Washington, their wives, and children offered themselves as subjects, and some of the private physicians, and in 1911, practically every garrison had been vaccinated.

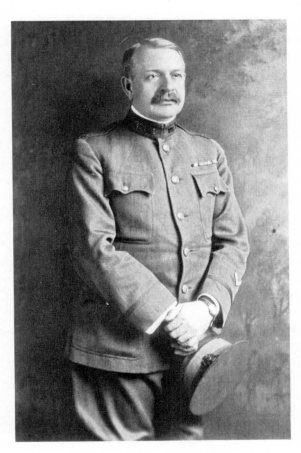

Not until the troops were mobilized in Texas for the manoeuvers, however, was the rule for vaccination with the antityphoid vaccine made compulsory. Sixty thousand doses were served to the troops in Texas and on the border, each man being inoculated three times, the entire treatment covering a period of twenty days. Although the soldiers mingled with the people of San Antonio and other cities where sanitary conditions were not always of the best in food supplies, water, or surroundings, and where typhoid prevailed as a general thing, there were few cases in the army, whereas in the Spanish-American War one-fourth to one-third of the men were

Frederick Russell (1870–1960). An American army physician, Russell tested and implemented a typhoid vaccination among American soldiers prior to the First World War (courtesy National Library of Medicine).

affected.... During the present year, with 58,000 troops, the largest number under experiment and used as comparison with any previous year, there were only 15 cases and 2 deaths from typhoid.

Only two physicians in the Army Medical School refused to be inoculated, and curiously enough they were the only two persons affected by typhoid during the school term.... The time had probably not yet come when this vaccination should be made compulsory throughout the country, but its use could be put into effect under certain conditions to the great[er] good to the community by local authorities in lumber camps, asylums, workhouses, almshouses, mines, and among travelers who were likely to be infected by conditions met with while away from home.... It would probably be many generations before this country would be as clear of typhoid as England and Germany.

Sanitary administration in this country has no national organization of force behind it to make it generally effective throughout the country. Many of the states have no sanitary system, and we see the doctrine of home rule in this respect carried to the point of absurdity.[21]

By the end of 1909 a total of 85 percent of the troops in the army had received the vaccine. In 1911 receipt of the typhoid vaccine became required for all members of the military. In combination with the use of proper sanitary procedures (chlorination of water was made standard practice in 1910 by Major Carl Rogers Darnell) mandatory vaccination resulted in the reduction of the incidence of typhoid among the troops from a high of some 14,000+ per 100,000 men, to that of 37 per 100,000 during World War 1. Even these numbers were somewhat misleading. Once the men were overseas in Europe they were subjected to conditions of water, food and milk contamination and inadequate sewage disposal in many of the areas in which they served. Not surprisingly, it was in these regions that exposure to the typhoid bacillus was much more frequent than it would have been back in the States. Chlorination of large quantities of water supplies was not always practical, or even possible. In addressing this problem, Major William Lyster, a member of the U.S. Army Medical Corps, developed in 1915 what became known as the Lyster bag, a linen bag containing calcium hypochlorite which could be used to purify water for drinking or other purposes. The bag was some 36" × 22" in size and could be hung from a tree or even a tent pole. After the bag was partially filled with water, a chlorine tablet was dropped into the water for purification. Faucets on the bottom allowed for dispersal of water. Initially used in World War I, the Lyster bag was utilized during the war in Vietnam.[22]

Typhoid fever was not the only enteric disease with which the army had to cope during these years. Paratyphoid fever is a similar, albeit milder, form of illness associated with infection by a different serotype of *Salmonella enterica*, the agent of typhoid. Two forms of paratyphoid fever were known at the time World War 1, types A and B. During September 1916 the Army Medical School released the first paratyphoid A vaccine, to be given in conjunction with the typhoid vaccine: three doses of typhoid vaccine and three doses of paratyphoid A vaccine. The following year the medical school released its trivalent vaccine containing inactivated typhoid bacilli as well as paratyphoid A and B; it was known as the TAB vaccine (triple typhoid saline vaccine). Since paratyphoid fever was relatively uncommon and inclusion of the paratyphoid strains appeared to reduce the efficacy of the typhoid vaccine, the paratyphoid B portion of the vaccine was removed in 1928 and the paratyphoid A portion in 1934.[23] The vaccine remained a monovalent one, containing only *Salmonella typhosa* (as the agent was then named) until the Second World War.

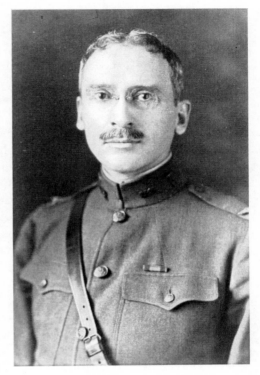

William Lyster (1869–1947). A member of the American Army Corps prior to the First World War, Lyster developed what became known as the Lyster bag, a filtration procedure for purification of water (courtesy National Library of Medicine).

During much of the decade of the Great Depression, particularly in the period from 1933 to 1939, it was the members of the Civilian Conservation Corps (CCC) who served as the epidemiological laboratory for the army. The CCC ultimately enrolled some 2.5 million youths who carried out their work throughout the United States. Employment in the CCC required vaccination against typhoid fever, a vaccination program overseen by the army. Despite immunization, a significant outbreak of typhoid fever occurred among the 195 men in a CCC camp near Ely, Minnesota, in December 1935. One hundred and forty of the men were with the CCC and had recently been vaccinated at Fort Leavenworth, Kansas, prior to leaving for Minnesota. Among the personnel at the camp were other workmen, most of whom had not been vaccinated.

Nearly everyone in the camp became ill, and eleven of the workmen died. All of the vaccinated men recovered. The camp had been located on a ledge of rock, with the camp water supply provided by a drilled well. Blasting operations had been carried out in the vicinity as the camp was being built and it was believed that in the process, fissures had opened in the rock, allowing effluent from latrines to enter the water supply from the well.[24]

The start of World War II is officially dated to September 1, 1939, when the German army invaded Poland. By mid–1940 most of western Europe had fallen to the German juggernaut, as well as portions of Asia to the Japanese. It was clear, at least in the mind of President Franklin Roosevelt, that it was only a matter of time before the United States would enter the war. If the United States entered the war it was likely that troops would be exposed to enteric organisms, including both the typhoid bacillus and the paratyphoid bacilli. On July 9, 1940, Surgeon General Thomas Parran, Jr., following the recommendation by a joint committee representing the army, navy and Public Health Service, ordered the commandant of the Army Medical School, Colonel George Callender, to resume the manufacture and use of the trivalent vaccine containing inactivated typhoid and paratyphoid A and B bacilli. The typhoid strain was the Panama carrier strain 58, chosen because of its ability to induce a maximum immune response as well as provide protection against other related strains with which troops might come into contact. When typhoid struck three American troops in India in 1942, this raised the question of cross-reactivity and whether additional strains of the typhoid bacillus should be used as well. However, it was determined that the India strain provided no better immunity in a vaccine than the Panama strain already in use.[25]

The efficacy of the trivalent vaccine can be clearly observed in the numbers. The combined annual rates for typhoid and paratyphoid A and B were on the order of 0.05 per thousand, a level which was one-eighth the rate for the combined diseases in the First World War (0.42 per thousand), itself a vast improvement from that in the Spanish-American War. Other diseases associated with contaminated water or food, such as dysentery, did not show comparable numbers, attesting as well to the effectiveness of the trivalent vaccine.

	Typhoid	Paratyphoid	Dysentery, diarrhea, enteritis
Total army	0.02	0.03	30.82
United States	0.01	0.01	19.97
Overseas	0.04	0.07	45.72[26]

Rates per 1000 of typhoid, paratyphoid A and B, and other diarrheal diseases

During World War II and in the immediate aftermath, the discovery and use of antibiotics in the treatment of infectious disease provided an effective means to control such illnesses. The most important of the first classes of antibiotics—penicillin and its derivatives and the sulfa drugs—were limited in their effectiveness in treating typhoid fever. The first antibiotic proven to be highly effective against typhoid fever, chloramphenicol, was discovered almost be chance.

Chloramphenicol was isolated during the 1940s by Dr. David Gottlieb from a strain of the bacterium *Streptomyces*. It was only after the war that this drug, dubbed chloromycetin by Parke, Davis and Company, its manufacturer, was widely applied. It was found to be highly efficacious against a broad spectrum of pathogenic bacteria including scrub typhus, the etiological agent of which is in a category known as Rickettsia. By chance, it was also found by army doctors to be effective in treating typhoid fever.

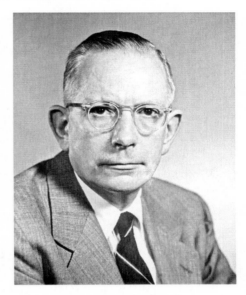

Joseph Smadel (1907–1963). An American physician and virologist, Smadel studied the use of antibiotics in treatment of typhoid and other bacterial diseases (courtesy National Library of Medicine).

In 1948, working under the auspices of the Walter Reed Army Medical Center, Drs. Joseph Smadel, Theodore Woodward and Herbert Ley were among those carrying out field studies in Kuala Lumpur, Malaysia, testing the newly developed drug chloromycetin in the treatment of the rickettsial disease epidemic typhus. By chance they observed that ten patients who were infected with typhoid also responded to treatment with the antibiotic.[27]

More extensive testing was carried out the following year in the United States by the Army Medical Department, the University of Maryland Medical School and the Commission on Immunization of the Army Epidemiological Board, comprised of Woodward, Smadel and Ley. Twenty-four patients "acutely ill" with typhoid fever and five typhoid carriers were treated with chloromycetin.[28] Treatment was begun with twenty-two of the patients within the first weeks after the illness began, while two patients were treated after a relapse of the disease that took place a month or two later. Individuals who received a full course of treatment recovered completely, while the patients who had suffered a relapse underwent lesser treatment at first. Once treatment with chloromycetin was resumed, these patients also recovered completely. Treatment of typhoid carriers was less successful, as four typhoid carriers continued to excrete the bacilli. As controls, other patients were treated with either the antibiotic aureomycin or the antibiotic polymyxin. Neither was successful in curing the illness. Other studies on the efficacy of chloromycetin in treating the carrier state showed comparable results—poor effectiveness in eliminating the organism from the patient.[29] For a time chloramphenicol became the drug of choice in treatment of typhoid fever. However, by the 1950s it was known that side effects were sometimes associated with use of the drug, including rare but often fatal cases of aplastic anemia. Strains of typhoid fever were also showing increasing resistance to the antibiotic. The development of other effective antibiotics in treatment of the disease meant chloramphenicol is today utilized only as a last resort. Nevertheless, the U.S. Army Medical Department had had pioneered the use of antibiotics in treating typhoid patients.

With the implementation of strict sanitation procedures and the development of new generations of typhoid vaccines (see Chapter 9) and antibiotics effective in treating the disease, typhoid fever had largely been eliminated as a problem for American service people by the new century. New recruits are still "subjected" to an extensive series of vaccinations, including those for rubella, measles, mumps, meningococcal infections, etc., with some variation among the services. Typhoid vaccination is no longer included, with the exception of those about to be deployed in areas in which the disease is endemic.[30] The current (2014) vaccination procedure for service members about to be deployed is similar to that recommended for civilians traveling to these areas:

a) Typhim Vi (Typhoid Vi Polysaccharide Vaccine) administered intramuscularly in the deltoid muscle, at least two weeks prior to potential exposure. A booster is recommended if it has been at least two years since a prior vaccination; or,

b) Vivotif (Typhoid Vaccine Live, Oral Ty21a), with four doses administered on alternate days, completed at least one week prior to potential exposure. A booster is recommended if prior vaccination with the oral version was more than five years earlier.[31]

12

Typhoid Fever in the 21st Century

Despite the nearly universal recognition that typhoid fever—or for that matter any foodborne or waterborne disease—is a problem generally associated with improper sanitation procedures, it remains a major challenge well into the 21st century. According to the statistics compiled by the Centers for Disease Control and Prevention (CDC) for the year 2000, the estimated worldwide incidence was some 22 million cases and over 200,000 deaths annually.[1] The morbidity numbers likely represent minimum values, with the actual incidence almost certainly significantly greater due to misdiagnosis and underreporting, as was illustrated in a 2010 study.[2] Those countries considered lowest on the socioeconomic scale would obviously be most at risk. For example, the highest reported incidence in 2010 was for the region of sub-Saharan Africa, averaging a minimum of 725 cases per 100,000 persons per year in 2010.[3] The actual incidence is likely even greater.

Several examples illustrate the challenges faced by healthcare workers. An outbreak in the Democratic Republic of Congo between September 2004 and the following January resulted in nearly 43,000 reported cases and over 200 deaths. As is frequently the case, the epidemic was the result of poor sanitary conditions and a lack of pure water for drinking or washing. The site in which many of these cases occurred was the capital city of Kinshasa. Since antibiotics continue to be the primary choice of therapy, once health care workers are available on the scene a major concern among physicians is the selection of resistant mutants among the typhoid bacilli. In an attempt to track possible development of resistant strains, between 2007 and 2011, physicians carried out a prospective study countrywide in which they tested samples of typhoid bacilli isolated from the bloodstreams of children and young adults for resistance against the most common forms of treatment. Multidrug-resistant strains were observed in nearly one-third of the isolates, posing a challenge for future attempts at control and containment.[4]

An outbreak in Delmas, South Africa, in 2005 resulted in over 600 diagnosed cases of typhoid fever. The strain which was isolated appeared identical to that which had caused a similar epidemic a decade earlier. Over 2,100 cases were diagnosed in the earlier outbreak. The source in both sets of cases was drinking water contaminated with fecal waste.[5] Even though no further outbreaks of similar size took place in South Africa during the rest of the decade, the disease has remained endemic in the region.

In portions of Southeast Asia such as India and Bangladesh, the annual incidence of typhoid was estimated at over 100 cases/100,000 persons in 2000.[6] More accurate figures are not readily available due to poor surveillance systems in those regions. There is no reason to think that the incidence is significantly different a decade later. India is a particular challenge, even given its progressive government and potential for proper health policies. We may be in the 21st century, but it is estimated that half of the citizens of India continue to defecate outdoors. Much of the sewage which is generated is untreated.[7] One could associate similar behaviors with the high incidence of disease found in other regions.

Given the modern understanding of the disease, several forms of intervention must be instituted in order to control the outbreaks in these regions. First is the need for improved access to properly treated drinking water, including, at a minimum, access to safe and clean water supplies. Second is the proper disinfection and disposal of fecal waste. An additional factor may be the institution of widespread vaccination in regions of the world in which typhoid is endemic. In 2008, similar means of control, in particular improved sanitation, were recommended by the World Health Organization (WHO). The organization also advocated increased access to, and use of, vaccines for any high-risk populations.[8]

Typhoid Fever in the United States

As a result of modern sanitation procedures, typhoid fever in the United States has largely been brought under control. During the 1920s, an estimated 35,000 cases were reported on an annual basis. The actual numbers were certainly greater. By the 1980s, the incidence was in the range of 300–400 cases per year, a number which has continued to decrease through the first decades of the twenty-first century. Most recent cases, an estimated 80 percent, have occurred in persons who had traveled during the two months preceding their illness to countries such as India, Mexico, the Philippines, Pakistan and Haiti, regions in which typhoid is endemic.[9] The remaining 20 percent of patients who were infected within the United States were exposed primarily through contaminated food or water, though in several cases the source may have been a healthy carrier. Several notable outbreaks were reported between 1975 and 2000. In 1981, 80 cases in Texas were attributed to a meal of steamed barbacoa, slow-cooked parts of a cow or sheep head, which had been prepared by a restaurant. In October and November of that same year, an outbreak occurred in Jackson, Michigan, among United Way workers who had attended a luncheon at a local banquet hall, sickening 18 of the 310 guests. The infections were believed to be linked to a food handler who was a typhoid carrier. A 1989 outbreak at a resort hotel in New York which affected 43 persons was the result of drinking contaminated orange juice. An additional two dozen cases were deemed probable but not confirmed. Two hotel employees were found to be typhoid carriers.

Most outbreaks between the year 2000 and the ensuing decade involved relatively small numbers, sometimes affecting different demographic groups. An outbreak of typhoid in 2000 in Indiana, Kentucky and Ohio involved seven gay men. The most recent reported epidemic was in the year 2012 and affected 12 persons in California and Nevada. The source was believed to be contaminated mamy fruit pulp imported from Guatemala.[10] While the incidence of typhoid in the United States remains relatively low, of particular concern are the increasing numbers of cases which have proven resistant to the most common forms of antibiotic treatment: ampicillin, chloramphenicol and trimethoprim-sulfamethoxazole.

In past decades, laboratory-acquired typhoid infections had been a problem, not only among the actual technicians handling such specimens but also in family members suffering from secondary exposure. Between 1977 and 1980, for example, 32 cases of laboratory-acquired typhoid fever were reported in the United States, a number which included two members of a microbiologist's family. There was one death.[11] Most of these cases were the result of carelessness on the part of the individual, either due to ingestion from mouth pipetting or contamination of hands or fingers and the subsequent transfer of organisms to the mouth. With stricter institution of aseptic procedures in the laboratory since then, such means of infection have been effectively eliminated.[12]

The significantly reduced incidence of typhoid fever in developed countries clearly shows control is possible. Unlike many diseases, both bacterial and viral, typhoid is found only in humans, meaning there is no non-human reservoir for the etiological agent. Nor is the United States the only developed country in which control has been established. In Israel, for example, the annual incidence was reduced from 90 per 100,000 during the 1950s to 0.23 per 100,000 by 2003. The reported incidence of the disease in developed countries as a whole during the early 21st century has been reduced to 0.13–1.2 cases per 100,000.[13]

As was noted above, most of the typhoid cases in developed countries do not originate within the region but are brought by travelers from areas in which the disease is endemic. Most of those cases originate in the Indian subcontinent, where the risk has been calculated as upwards of 18 times that of any other region.[14]

Treatment and Prevention in the 21st Century

The discovery and development of antibiotics in the years following World War II resulted in an effective means to treat most bacterial diseases, including typhoid. Three antibiotics in particular—chloramphenicol, ampicillin and trimethoprim-sulfamethoxazole—were particularly useful. However, as alluded to above, by the 1980s and 1990s strains of *Salmonella* resistant to the antibiotics were beginning to appear. In some cases, the means of resistance was acquired through the transfer of plasmids, small independent pieces of DNA passed among bacteria. Often this genetic material contained multiple genes which conferred resistance to several antibiotics simultaneously, even when the recipient bacterium had not been exposed to all of these drugs. The development of a new class of antibiotics, the fluoroquinolones, alleviated the problem of resistance for a time. However, new strains resistant to this class as well began to appear. The problems inherent in this situation are obvious. The presence of resistant strains results in slower and less effective forms of treatment. This does not even take into account the significant increase in cost in treating such infections, a burden that less developed countries can ill afford.

The other preventive option in endemic regions is the typhoid vaccine. Currently, two forms of the vaccine are in use. The live vaccine, Ty21a, is an attenuated form of the bacillus lacking the Vi (virulence) surface antigen. Its development was described in a previous chapter. While this vaccine can be administered orally, it does have several drawbacks. Since the organism is alive, it cannot be administered to individuals already on antibiotic therapy. For optimal efficacy, three to four doses are also required. The alternative vaccine consists of the purified surface polysaccharide, the Vi antigen. It is administered as an injection, but the fact that it consists of a polysaccharide rather than protein limits its ability to induce a long-term immune response. A modified form of the vaccine in which the Vi antigen is chemically attached to a protein carrier, already in use in endemic countries, should help address this shortcoming in the future.

Of course, the most effective way to control typhoid in the future is to prevent its spread in the first place. But, as with the situation with drug therapy in economically depressed countries, the cost to invest in the education and development of infrastructure necessary to control such diseases is often too much for these governments.

Chapter Notes

Preface

1. George Chandler Whipple, *Typhoid Fever: Its Causation, Transmission and Prevention* (New York: John Wiley & Sons, 1908), xxv.

2. Burke A. Cunha, "Osler on Typhoid Fever: Differentiating Typhoid from Typhus and Malaria," *Infectious Disease Clinics of North America* 18 (2004): 111–125.

3. Arthur Allen, *The Fantastic Laboratory of Dr. Weigl* (New York: W.W. Norton, 2014), 20.

4. Celsus, *De Medicina*, Book 3, Loeb Classical Library (Cambridge: Harvard University Press, 1997), cited by Cheston B. Cunha, "Prolonged and Perplexing Fevers in Antiquity: Malaria and Typhoid Fever," *Infectious Disease Clinics of North America* 21 (2007): 857–866.

5. Victor C. Vaughan, Henry F. Vaughan and George T. Palmer, "The Typhoid Fevers," in *Epidemiology and Public Health*, vol. 2 (St. Louis: C.V. Mosby, 1923), 268–270.

6. Cunha, *op. cit.*, 864.

7. Manolis J. Papagrigorakis, Christos Yapijakis and Philippos N. Synodinos, "Typhoid Fever Epidemic in Ancient Athens," in *Paleomicrobiology: Past Human Infections*, ed. D. Raoult and M. Drancourt (Berlin: Springer-Verlag, 2008), 161–173.

8. David L. Grove, *Tapeworms, Lice and Prions: A Compendium of Unpleasant Infections* (New York: Oxford University Press, 2014), 327.

9. Thomas Willis, "Of a Putrid Feaver," in *Classic Descriptions of Disease,* ed. Ralph Major (IL: Charles C. Thomas, 1945), 179–181.

10. W.C. Summers, "Typhoid, historical," in *Encyclopedia of Microbiology*, 2nd ed. (New York: Academic Press, 2000), 97.

11. Cunha, "Osler," 112.

12. North British Agriculturalist, "Contagious Diseases," *American Farmer: A Monthly Magazine of Agriculture and Horticulture* 2 (1868), 43.

13. W. Osler, *The Principles and Practice of Medicine*, 8th ed. (London: Appleton, 1919).

14. D.E. Salmon and T. Smith, "Report on Swine Plague," *U.S. Bureau of Animal Industries: 2nd Annual Report* (Washington, D.C.: U.S. Government Printing Office, 1885).

15. James H. Steele, "Epidemiology of Salmonellosis," *Public Health Reports* 78, no. 12 (December 1963): 1065–1066.

16. H. Laude, "Isolation of a Cytolytic Strain of Hog Cholera Virus from IB-RS2 Cells," *Annals of Microbiology* 129, no. 4 (Paris) (May–June 1978): 553–561.

17. Theobald Smith, Special Report on the Cause and Prevention of Swine Plague (Washington, D.C.: Government Printing Office, 1891), 15–16.

Chapter 1

1. Cited by Matthew L. Lim and Mark R. Wallace, "Infectious Diarrhea in History," *Infectious Disease Clinics of North America* 18 (2004): 261–274; Karen Dixon and Pat Southern, *The Roman Cavalry* (New York: Routledge, 1997), 94.

2. H. Curschmann, *Typhoid Fever and Typhus Fever*, ed. William Osler (translated under the editorial supervision of Alfred

Stengel, M.D.) (Philadelphia: W.B. Saunders, 1901), 17.

3. http://www.perseus.tufts.edu/hop per/text?doc=Perseus:text:1999.01.,0251: text=intro.

4. Hippocrates, *The Genuine Works of Hippocrates*, vol. 1, translated from the Greek by Francis Adams, LLD (London: Sydenham Society, 1849).

5. Dark urine is not necessarily typical of typhoid. However, if the patient was dehydrated, as suggested by the dry tongue, the concentrated urine may have appeared dark.

6. Hippocrates, *Genuine Works*, 371–372.

7. *Ibid.*, 376. The pouring of hot water over the head was a method of treatment for fever recommended by Hippocrates.

8. William Henry Welch, *Papers and Addresses by William Henry Welch*, vol. 1 (Baltimore: Johns Hopkins University Press, 1920), 463.

9. Victor C. Vaughan, Henry F. Vaughan and George T. Palmer, *Epidemiology and Public Health*, vol. 2 (St. Louis: C.V. Mosby, 1923), 263.

10. Herodotus, *The Histories*, trans. George Rawlinson (digireads.com publishing, 2009), 344–345; also cited by Lim, 263.

11. http://www.poetryintranslation.com/ PITBR/Latin/Suetonius2.htm#_Toc276121 9.21; Suetonius, *The Twelve Caesars*, Book II, *Augustus* LIX, "Offerings and Commemorations," (A.S. Kline (translation), 2010); Patricia Southern, *Augustus*, 2nd ed. (New York: Routledge, 2014), 203–204.

12. Fielding H. Garrison, *An Introduction to the History of Medicine* (Philadelphia: W.B. Saunders, 1922), 178–179.

13. *Ibid.*, 181; Karl Sudhoff, "The Origin of Syphilis," *Bulletin of the Society of Medical History of Chicago* 2, no. 1 (January 1917): 17–18.

14. http://www.fofweb.com/History/ MainPrintPage.asp?iPin=ENPP205&Data Type=WorldHistory.

15. Samuel Cooper, "Lectures on the Principles, Practices and Operations of Surgery," *London Medical and Surgical Journal* 4, no. 98 (December 14, 1833): 614.

16. Sudhoff, "Origin of Syphilis."

17. Garrison, *Introduction to History of Medicine*, n181; "Febris Gallica, epidemia" *Bibliotheca Medico-Practica* (Geneva: Haeredum Cramer & Fratrum Philibert, 1739), 824.

18. Garrison, *Introduction to History of Medicine*.

Chapter 2

1. Thucydides, *The History of the Peloponnesian War*, Book 2, chapter 7, pp. 2.47–2.55.

2. *Ibid.*, 2.48.1.

3. Burke A. Cunha, "The Cause of the Plague of Athens: Plague, Typhoid, Typhus, Smallpox or Measles?" *Infectious Disease Clinics of North America* 18, no. 1 (March 2004): 29–43.

4. *Ibid.*

5. Thucydides, *History of the War.*

6. *Ibid.*, also cited by Arthur M. Silverstein and Alexander A. Bialasiewicz, "History of Immunology: A History of Acquired Immunity," *Cellular Immunology* 51 (1980): 151–167.

7. S. Sarasombath et al., "Systemic and Intestinal Immunities After Natural Typhoid Infection," *Journal of Clinical Microbiology* 25, no. 6 (June 1987): 1088–1093.

8. David T. Durack, Robert J. Littman, R. Michael Benitez and Philip A. Mackowiak, "Hellenic Holocaust: A Historical Clinico-Pathologic Conference," *American Journal of Medicine* 109, no. 8 (October 1, 2000): 391–397.

9. *Ibid.*

10. Manolis Papagrigorakis et al., "Typhoid Epidemic in Ancient Athens," 161–173, in D. Raoult and M. Drancourt, ed., *Paleomicrobiology: Past Human Infections* (Berlin: Springer-Verlag, 2008).

11. D. Raoult et al., "Molecular Identification by Suicide PCR of *Yersinia pestis* as the Agent of Medieval Black Death," *Proceedings of the National Academy of Sciences USA* 97, no. 23 (November 7, 2000): 12800–12803.

12. *Ibid.*

13. Durack, "Hellenic Holocaust," 396.

Chapter 3

1. Plutarch, *Lives*, vol. 7 (Cambridge, MA: Harvard University Press, 1958), 241. Stageira was conquered and destroyed by Philip in 348 BCE during the military campaign.

2. *Ibid.*, 251.

3. *Ibid.*, 349–351.

4. *Ibid.*, 357.

5. *Ibid.*, 433.

6. http://hellenspot.narod.ru/page3. htm; A.B. Bosworth, "The Death of Alexander the Great: Rumour and Propaganda," *Classical Quarterly* 21 (1971): 112–136. There are few known contemporary references to Ephippus. According to Arrian in his work written a half century later, Ephippus had been appointed by Alexander as one of his administrators in Egypt. As a source for the 12-pint cup, Ephippus is questionable (Andrew Chugg, *The Quest for the Tomb of Alexander the Great* [AMC, 2007], 239).

7. http://penelope.uchicago.edu/Thayer/E/Roman/Texts/Diodorus_Siculus/17F*.html; Bill Thayer, *The Library of History of Diodorus Siculus*, Loeb Classic Library ed., vol. 8, Book 17 (1963), 467. In a footnote, Thayer explained the "cup of Heracles" as a commemoration of the death of Heracles on Mt. Oeta, an event with which Medius would have been "familiar."

8. Plutarch, *Lives*, 433–435.

9. E.J. Chinnock, *The Anabasis of Alexander; or, The History of the Wars and Conquests of Alexander the Great*, "Literally Translated, with a Commentary, from the Greek of Arrian the Nicomedian" (London: Hodder and Stoughton, 1884), 418–420.

10. Cunha, "The Death of Alexander the Great," *Infectious Disease Clinics of North America* 18 (2004): 53–63; Philip A. Mackowiak, *Post Mortem* (Philadelphia: American College of Physicians, 2007), 59–82.

11. Cunha, "The Death of Alexander," 58.

12. David Oldach, Robert Richard, Eugene Borza and R. Michael Benitez, "A Mysterious Death," *New England Journal of Medicine* 338, no. 24 (June 11, 1998): 1764–1769.

13. Mackowiak, *op. cit.*

14. Plutarch, *Lives*, 425.

Chapter 4

1. Much of the terminology used in the sciences has its origins in nineteenth century and early twentieth century Austria-Hungary and Germany, then among the centers of scientific research. The nomenclature of O and H antigens used today to designate bacterial structures may have had its origin with Edmund Weil and Arthur Felix in the first decades of the twentieth century. When studying the highly motile enteric organism *Proteus*, Weil and Felix observed a characteristic spreading film on the surface of an agar plate which they had inoculated. Its similarity to breath resulted in the designation of *Hauch*. Strains which were not motile were "without breath," *Ohne Hauch.* The designations of O and H were subsequently applied to the somatic and flagellar antigens, respectively. "Capsule" in German was spelled with a K.

2. Pushpa Maurya, Anil K. Gulati and Gopal Nath, "Status of Vi Gene, Its Expression and Salmonella Pathogenicity Island (SPI-7) in *Salmonella typhi* in India," *Southeast Asian Journal of Tropical Medicine and Public Health* 41, no. 4 (July 2010): 913–919. What is referred to as a pathogenicity island is a mobile region found in many bacteria which encode genes contributing to the pathogenicity of an organism. As many as fifteen such "islands" have been identified in the *Salmonella* genome in various serovars.

3. John Wain et al., "Vi Antigen Expression in *Salmonella enterica* Serovar typhi Clinical Isolates from Pakistan," *Journal of Clinical Microbiology* 43, no. 3 (March 2005): 1158–1165.

4. R.J. Looney and R.T. Steigbigel, "Role of the Vi Antigen in *Salmonella typhi* in resistance to host defense in vitro," *Journal of Laboratory and Clinical Medicine* 108, no. 5 (November 1986): 506–516.

5. *Ibid.*

6. Amin Tahoum et al., "*Salmonella* Transforms Follicle-Associated Epithelial Cells into M Cells to Promote Intestinal Invasion," *Cell Host and Microbe* 12, no. 5 (November 2012): 607–609.

7. Bradley Jones, Hugh F. Paterson, Alan Hall and Stanley Falkow, "*Salmonella typhimurium* induces membrane ruffling by a growth-factor-independent mechanism," *Proceedings of the National Academy of Sciences USA* 90 (November 1993): 10390–10394.

8. S.R. Waterman and D.W. Holden, "Functions and effectors of the *Salmonella* pathogenicity island 2 type III secretion system," *Cellular Microbiology* 5, no. 8 (August 2003): 501–511.

9. Robert W. Crawford et al., "Gallstones Play a Significant Role in *Salmonella* spGallbladder Colonization and Carriage," *Proceedings of the National Academy of Sciences USA* 107, no. 9 (March 2, 2010): 4353–4358.

10. *Ibid.*

11. John Gunn, "Mechanisms of Bacter-

ial Resistance and Response to Bile," *Microbes and Infection* 2, no. 8 (July 2000): 907–913.

12. Dijun Du et al., "Structure of the AcrAB-TolC Multidrug Efflux Pump," *Nature* 509 (May 22, 2014): 512–515.

13. Gunn, *op. cit.*

14. *Ibid.*

15. E.A. Groisman, "The Pleiotropic Two-component Regulatory System PhoP-PhoQ," *Journal of Bacteriology* 183, no. 6 (March 2001): 1835–1842.

16. A.M. Prouty and J.S. Gunn, "*Salmonella enterica* serovar Typhimurium Invasion Is Repressed in the Presence of Bile," *Infection and Immunity* 68, no. 12 (December 2000): 6763–6769.

17. Hyunjin Yoon, Charles Ansong, Joshua N. Adkins and Fred Heffron, "Discovery of *Salmonella* Virulence Factors Translocated Via Outer Membrane Vesicles to Murine Macrophage," *Infection and Immunity* 79, no. 6 (June 2011): 2182–2192.

18. Salih Hosoglu et al., "Risk Factors for Enteric Perforation in Patients with Typhoid Fever," *American Journal of Epidemiology* 160, no. 1 (July 1, 2004): 46–50.

19. Jasmine Kaur and S.K. Jain, "Role of Antigens and Virulence Factors of *Salmonella enterica* serovar Typhi in Its Pathogenesis," *Microbiological Research* 167 (2012): 199–210. A much more detailed listing of additional effector proteins may be found in the source.

20. *Ibid.*

Chapter 5

1. Edward Percival, "Practical Observations on the Treatment, Pathology and Prevention of Typhus Fever," *London Medical Repository, Monthly Journal and Review* 11, no. 64 (April 1, 1819): 398.

2. Leonard Wilson, "Fevers," in *Companion Encyclopedia of the History of Medicine,* ed. W.F. Bynum and Roy Porter (London: Routledge, 1993), 398. Peruvian bark, also known as Jesuit's bark, was a common medicinal used in the treatment of malaria (and other fevers) because of its high content of quinine.

3. William Budd, *On the Causes of Fevers* (1839), ed. Dale Smith (Baltimore: Johns Hopkins University Press, 1984).

4. *Ibid.*, 6.

5. Thomas Willis, "Of a Putrid Fever,"

in Ralph Major, *Classic Descriptions of Disease,* 3rd ed. (Springfield, IL: Charles Thomas, 1945), 179–182.

6. Fielding Garrison, *An Introduction to the History of Medicine* (Philadelphia: W.B. Saunders, 1922), 262; Major, 238.

7. http://www.whonamedit.com/doctor.cfm/336.html.

8. W.C. Summers, "Typhoid, Historical," in *Encyclopedia of Microbiology*, ed. Moselio Schaechter (San Diego: Elsevier/Academic, 2009), 97. As an interesting sidelight, in 1787 Dr. Erasmus Darwin presented a question to the Royal Society as to "whether the nervous fever of Huxham be the same as the petechial or jail fever." Jail fever was likely typhus. While Erasmus Darwin was well known in his own right, he is also famous as the grandfather of the naturalist Charles Darwin (Charles Murchison, *A Treatise on the Continued Fevers of Great Britain,* 3rd ed. [London: Longmans, Green, 1884], 424).

9. Murchison, 423.

10. *Ibid.* Gilchrist (1707–1774) was noted for his use of treatments utilized by ancient physicians, including wine and warm baths. He was also among those advocating variolation as a means of protection against smallpox.

11. *Ibid.* Langrish (d. 1759) was known for his studies in muscular motion as well as metabolic byproducts found in feces.

12. Jacques-Rene Tenon, *Mémoire sur les hôpitaux de Paris* [Memoirs on the Hospitals of Paris], 1788), quoted by Erwin Ackernecht at www.mini4stroke.tweakdsl.nl/Histmedsc/Ackerknecht.pdf (16).

13. Ackernacht, 19.

14. *Ibid.*, 3.

15. *Ibid.*, 4.

16. *Ibid.*, 6.

17. *Ibid.*, 9.

18. W.H. Corfield, "The Milroy Lectures on the Etiology of Typhoid Fever and Its Prevention," *Lancet* 159, no. 4099 (March 22, 1902): 793–803; de Hildenbrand, Johann Valentin, trans. S.D. Gross, *A Treatise on the Nature, Cause, and Treatment of Contagious Typhus* (New York: Elam Bliss, 1829). The authors would also like to clarify the nobiliary designations "von" or "de" (of): "von" would be used in the original German; "de" is used in English translations.

19. von Hildenbrand, *ibid.*, 77.

20. Budd, *op. cit.*, 13–14.

21. *Ibid.*, 14.

22. Murchison, *op. cit.*, 426. There are several variations in spelling of the term "dothinenenteritis." We have used the spelling as found in the source.

23. Budd, *op. cit.*, 15.

24. *Ibid.*, 14; M. Trousseau, "Concerning the Disease to Which M. Bretonneau, Physician of the Hospital of Tours, Has Given the Name of Dothinenteritis," in Major, *op. cit.*, 182–184.

25. R. Heller, "Officiers de Santé," *Medical History* 22, no.1 (January 1978): 25–43. In the years immediately following the French Revolution, universities and medical societies were largely abolished. Because of the need for properly trained medical personnel, examination boards were established for regulation of the practice of medicine. Persons titled as doctors or surgeons were required to possess certain qualifications. The position of "officier de santé," albeit at a lower level, still required passing an examination administered by a board.

26. Major, *op. cit.*, 157–159. Bretonneau's choice of terminology was criticized by François Broussais, a physician on the faculty in Paris as meaning "inflammation of a skin." Knowing his Greek, Bretonneau responded with the explanation that the "itis" did not necessarily refer to inflammation. In this case it served as a noun, and diphtheritis represented a specific disease. The modern term for the disease is diphtheria.

27. P.C.A. Louis, "*Recherches anatomiques…*," in Major, 186–187. A second edition was published in 1841. Both editions were dedicated to Dr. Auguste-François Chomel, professor of clinical medicine at the university in Paris where he served as chair of that department. Chomel likewise considered typhus and typhoid to be separate and unique diseases: "We shall preferably call it by the name of typhoid fever or disease, because of the analogy which it offers in its symptoms with the typhus of camps" (1834) (Corfield, *op. cit.*, 796).

28. Budd, *op. cit.*, 16.

29. Corfield, *op. cit.*, 796.

30. *Ibid.*

31. Harris L. Coulter, *Divided Legacy: A History of the Schism in Medical Thought* (Berkeley, CA: North Atlantic Books, 2000), 517. Gendron likewise recognized that recovery from an attack protected the individual against a recurrence of the same illness. He replaced the term *accoutumance* (habituation) *with immunité* (immunity) in describing this phenomenon. He also used the phrase incubation period to indicate the period of time between exposure and the infectious period.

32. Corfield, *op. cit.*

33. David McCullough, *The Greater Journey, Americans in Paris* (New York: Simon & Schuster, 2011), 123.

34. John G. Simmons, "Pierre Louis: The Numerical Method," in *Doctors and Discoveries: Lives That Created Today's Medicine* (Boston: Houghton Mifflin, 2002), 275–276.

35. *Ibid.*, 276.

36. *Ibid.* In 1816 Laennec (1781–1826) developed the stethoscope, the use of which he applied in diagnosis of tuberculosis. Ironically Laennec himself died from that disease at the age of 45.

37. McCullough, *op cit.*, 12.

38. Alfred Hudson, *Lectures on the Study of Fever* (Philadelphia: Henry C. Lea, 1869), 275–277; Reprint of report by Bright in *Medical Reports* 1, p. 180; Budd, 13.

39. Budd, *op. cit.*, 13.

40. H.C. Lombard, *Dublin Journal of Medical Science* 10, no. 28 (September 1836): 17–24. Dr. Robert James Graves, who described the eponymously named Graves' disease, was a prominent Irish endocrinologist of the time. Among Graves' interests was the study of typhus, which makes it likely this was the person to whom Lombard's letters were directed.

41. *Ibid.*, 101–105; Elisha Bartlett, *The History, Diagnosis and Treatment of Typhoid and of Typhus Fever* (Philadelphia: Lea and Blanchard, 1842), 287–288.

42. W.W. Gerhard, "On the Typhus Fever Which Occurred at Philadelphia in the Spring and Summer of 1836, illustrated by Clinical Observations, Showing the Distinction Between This Form of Disease and Dothinenteritis or Typhoid Fever," *American Journal of Medical Sciences* 19 (1837): 289–291, 294, 307.

43. William Jenner, *On the Identity or Non-Identity of the Specific Cause of Typhoid, Typhus and Relapsing Fever* (London: John Churchill, 1850), 2.

44. *Ibid.*, 100.

45. Jenner, William, "On the Identity or Non-Identity of the Specific Cause of

Typhoid, Typhus and Relapsing Fever," *Transactions of the Royal Medical and Chirurgical Society* 33 (1850): 23–42.

46. William Budd, *On the Causes of Fevers* (1839), ed. Dale Smith (Baltimore: Johns Hopkins University Press, 1984), 9.

47. *Ibid.*, 49.

48. *Ibid.*, 30.

49. *Ibid.*, 3. Budd did not win, the award being presented to William Davidson, a physician of the Glasgow Royal Infirmary. Davidson's contention was that typhoid and typhus were different manifestations of the same disease (Budd, 33). The prize was awarded only that once.

50. Robert Moorhead, "William Budd and Typhoid Fever," *Journal of the Royal Society of Medicine* 95, no. 11 (November 2002): 561–564.

51. Budd, 76–77.

52. Moorhead. The building was destroyed during the German blitz in 1940.

53. *Ibid.*

54. William Budd, *Typhoid Fever: Its Nature, Mode of Spreading, and Prevention* (London: Longmans, Green, 1873), 128–135.

55. *Ibid.*, 136–138.

56. Moorhead, *op. cit.*

57. Robert Dorfman, Henry Jacoby and Harold Thomas, *Models for Managing Regional Water Quality* (Cambridge, MA: Harvard University Press, 1972), 3.

58. Budd, *op. cit.*, 161–162.

Chapter 6

1. Gillian Gill, *We Two: Victoria and Albert, Rulers, Partners, Rivals* (Ballantine, 2009), 161.

2. *Ibid.*, 24–31.

3. *Ibid.*, 130.

4. *Ibid.*, 132.

5. Jane Ridley, *The Heir Apparent: A Life of Edward VII, the Playboy Prince* (New York: Random House, 2014), 68–71.

6. *Ibid.*, 69–70.

7. *Ibid.*, 73.

8. Gill, *op. cit.*, 363.

9. "The Death of the Prince Consort," *Lancet* 2, no. 25 (December 21, 1861): 599–600; "Death of the Prince Consort: The Illness and Last Moments of the Prince," *London Observer*, December 23, 1861, p. 5.

10. Ridley, *op. cit.*, 75.

11. Gillian Gill, *We Two: Victoria and Albert, Rulers, Partners, Rivals* (Ballantine,

2009), 346–363; Christopher Hibbert, *Queen Victoria: A Personal History* (Cambridge, MA: Da Capo, 2001); Stanley Weintraub, *Victoria* (New York: E. Dutton, 1988), 293–301.

12. *Ibid.*, 359.

13. *Lancet, op. cit.*

14. *Ibid.*

15. Weintraub, *op. cit.*, 300.

16. R.O. Tilden, "Twentieth Century Plumbing," *Plumbers Trade Journal* 32, no. 1 (July 1, 1902: 58–60, cites letters from the Marquise de Fontenoy (pseudonym of Marguerite Owen); Marquise de Fontenoy, "Ill Health in Royal Palaces," *Washington Post*, November 19, 1900, p. 6.

17. Ridley, *op. cit.*, 182–187.

18. Weintraub, *op. cit.*, 371.

19. "Report of the Lancet Sanitary Commission on the State of Londesborough Lodge and Sandringham, in Relation to the Illness of H.R.H. The Prince of Wales," *Lancet*, December 9, 1871, pp. 828–831.

20. *Ibid.*

21. *Ibid.*

22. Stephen Ashwal, "William Gerhard," in *The Founders of Child Neurology*. Edited by Stephen Ashwal (San Francisco: Norman, 1990), 122.

23. William Jenner, "On the Identity or Non-Identity of the Specific Cause of Typhoid, Typhus and Relapsing Fever," *Edinburgh Monthly Journal of Medical Medicine* (April 1849); "On the Identity and Non-Identity of the Specific Cause of Typhoid, Typhus and Relapsing Fever," *Medico-Chirurgical Transactions* 33 (1850): 23–42.

24. "Obituary, Sir William Jenner," *British Medical Journal* 2, no. 1981 (December 17, 1898): 1849–1853.

25. *Ibid.*

26. Jane McHugh and Philip A. Mackowiak, "Death in the White House: President William Henry Harrison's Atypical Pneumonia," *Clinical Infectious Diseases* (Advance Access) (July 29, 2014), 1–6.

27. Thomas Miller, "Case of the Late William H. Harrison, President of the United States," *Boston Medical and Surgical Journal* 24, no. 17 (June 2, 1841): 261–267.

28. *Ibid.*

29. McHugh and Mackowiak, *op. cit.*

30. Robert J. Scarry, *Millard Fillmore* (Jefferson, NC: McFarland, 2001), 153.

31. K. Jack Bauer, *Zachary Taylor: Soldier,*

Planter, Statesman of the Old Southwest (Baton Rouge: Louisiana State University Press, 1985), 314–316.

32. http://web.ornl.gov/info/ornlreview/rev27–12/text/ansside6.html.

33. http://www.dailykos.com/story/2005/05/29/117856/-THE-STRANGE-DEATH-OF-ZACHARY-TAYLOR#.

34. http://www.politico.com/news/stories/0611/57126.html.

Chapter 7

1. Roy Porter, *The Greatest Benefit to Mankind: A Medical History of Humanity* (New York: W.W. Norton, 1997), 407. Educated as a physician, Villermé became better known as an economist and moralist.

2. *Ibid.*, 408.

3. *Ibid.*, 411–412.

4. Charles Murchison, *A Treatise on the Continued Fevers of Great Britain.* 2nd ed. (London: Longmans, Green, 1873), 660.

5. *Ibid.*, 10–11.

6. *Ibid.*, 12.

7. Steere-Williams, "The Perfect Food and the Filth Disease: Milk-borne Typhoid and Epidemiological Practice in Late Victorian England," *Journal of the History of Medicine* 65, no. 4 (March 2010): 514–545.

8. *Ibid.*, 522–524.

9. *Ibid.*, 537.

10. *Ibid.*, 538.

11. Gerald Geison, *The Private Science of Louis Pasteur* (Princeton, NJ: Princeton University Press, 1995), 36.

12. *Ibid.*, 113.

13. *Ibid.*, 124.

14. *Ibid.*, 125.

15. *Ibid.*, 120.

16. *Ibid.*, 22–24.

17. *Ibid.*, 30–31.

18. Geison's is arguably the most complete and detailed of the Pasteur biographies. René Dubos's *Louis Pasteur: Free Lance of Science* (New York: Da Capo, 1960) was the classic of its day. Dubos (1901–1982), professor emeritus of microbiology at the Rockefeller Institute, placed the story in the context of the times. Both biographies are excellent reads on the subject.

19. Geison, *op. cit.*, 148.

20. Thomas Gage, "The Prevention of the Spread of Typhoid Fever," *Medical Communications of the Massachusetts Medical Society* 12, no. 1 (1875): 353–388, 370–371.

21. *Ibid.*, 376.

22. Thomas Brock, *Robert Koch: A Life in Medicine and Bacteriology* (Washington, D.C.: American Society for Microbiology, 1999), 31.

23. *Ibid.*

24. *Ibid.*, 32.

25. *Ibid.*, 99.

26. *Ibid.*, 36.

27. *Ibid.*, 49.

28. *Ibid.*, 29.

29. *Ibid.*, 179. Loeffler and Klebs are credited with isolation and identification of the etiological agent of diphtheria, now known as *Corynebacterium diphtheriae.*

30. *Ibid.*, 11; http://www.encyclopedia.com/topic/Robert_Koch.aspx.

31. http://www.encyclopedia.com/topic/Robert_Koch.aspx.

32. Brock, *ibid.*, 14.

33. *Ibid.*, 20.

34. J. Stachura and K. Galazka, "History and Current Status of Polish Gastroenterological Pathology," *Journal of Physiology and Pharmacology* 54, no. 3 (2003: 183–192. The inability or lack of opportunity to associate the organisms he observed with typhoid correctly prevented Borowicz from receiving credit for his discovery. It would appear another oversight prevented credit for discovery of the Kuppfer cells in the liver being assigned to Browicz. Credit for discovery of the eponymously named phagocytic cells was given to the German anatomist Karl Kuppfer, who in 1876 described the presence of star-shaped cells (*sternzelle*) in that organ. At approximately the same time, Browicz described a set of oblong cells in the lumen of the liver. It appears that what Kuppfer had described were not the phagocytic cells from the organ but perisinusoidal cells, which store vitamin A. Browicz may have discovered the actual phagocytes (Andrzej Śródka et al., "Browicz or Kuppfer Cells?" [*Polish Journal of Pathology*] 57, no. 4 [2006]: 183–185).

35. David Grove, *Tapeworms, Lice and Prions: A Compendium of Unpleasant Infections* (New York: Oxford University Press, 2014), 332.

36. Frederick Parker Gay, *Typhoid Fever Considered as a Problem of Scientific Medicine* (New York: Macmillan, 1918), 8.

37. *Ibid.*

38. Grove, *op. cit.*

39. Gay, *op. cit.*, 9.

Chapter 8

1. Hermann Biggs and William H. Park, "The Serum-Test for the Diagnosis of Typhoid Fever," *American Journal of the Medical Sciences* 113, no. 3 (March 1897): 274–297.

2. Arthur M. Silverstein, "History of Immunology: Cellular Versus Humoral Immunity: Determinants and Consequences of an Epic 19th Century Battle," *Cellular Immunology* 48 (1979): 208–221.

3. *Ibid.*

4. G. Nuttall, "Experimente über die bacterienfeindlichen Einflüsse des theirischen Körpers," *Zeitschrift für Hygiene* 4 (1888): 353–95.

5. R. Pfeiffer, "Weitere Untersuchungen über das Wesen der cholera immunitat und über specifische bactericide process," *Zeitschrift für Hygiene* 18 (1894): 1–16.

6. Silverstein, *op. cit.*, 215.

7. *Medical News* 68 (May 9, 1896): 19.

8. http://www.aim25.ac.uk/cats/37/8112.htm.

9. M. Gruber, "Theorie der active und passive Immunitat gegen Cholera, Typhus und verwandte Krankheits processe," *Münchener medicinische Wochenschrift* 43, no. 9 (1896): 206.

10. Biggs and Park, *op. cit.*, 275.

11. [Richard] Pfeiffer and [Wilhelm] Kolle, "The Differential Diagnosis of Typhoid Fever by Means of the Serum of Animals Immunized Against Typhoid Infection," *Deutsche medicinische Wochenschrift* (March 1896): 12; Charles Frederick Bolduan and John Koopman, *Immune Sera: A Concise Exposition of Our Present Knowledge of Infection and Immunity* (New York: John Wiley, 1917), 53. Kolle by 1896 was a member of the Berlin Institute, where he carried out his typhoid research while working with Pfeiffer. His presence there had an element of serendipity. It appears Koch in his youth had fallen in love with a young woman whose family disapproved of the future physician and bacteriologist. The woman subsequently married someone else with the surname Kolle. When their son Wilhelm demonstrated an interest in bacteriology, the mother contacted Koch, asking for help in securing young Wilhelm a position. In 1893 Kolle joined the Institute (Pauline Mazumdar, *Species and Specificity* (New York: Cambridge University Press, 1995), 93).

12. Biggs and Park, *op. cit.*, 275–276.

13. Gruber, *op. cit.*; *Wiener Klinische Wochenschrift* (1896), Nos. 11, 12; cited by Biggs and Park, *op. cit.*

14. Herbert E. Durham, "A Special Action of the Serum of Highly Immunized Animals and Its Use for Diagnostic and Other Purposes," *Proceedings of the Royal Society* 59 (January 23, 1896), 355; *British Medical Journal* (Abstract), *Epitome of Medical Literature* (March 14, 1896): 44; *New York Medical Journal* 63, no. 16 (1896: 143–144); also cited by Biggs and Park, *op. cit.*, 277.

15. Herbert E. Durham, "Note on the Diagnostic Value of the Serum of Typhoid Fever Patients," *Lancet* 148, no. 3825 (December 19, 1896): 1746.

16. *Ibid.*

17. William Henry Welch, "Serum Diagnosis of Typhoid Fever," *Papers and Addresses*, vol. 2, *Bacteriology* (Baltimore: Johns Hopkins University Press, 1920), 352.

18. P. Horton-Smith, "The Goulstonian Lectures on the Typhoid Bacillus and Typhoid Fever," *Lancet* 1, no. 3996 (April 14, 1900): 1050–1063.

19. Henri Roger, *Infectious Diseases: Their Etiology, Diagnosis and Treatment* (New York: Lea Brothers, 1903), 559.

20. J. Bordet, *Annales de l'institut Pasteur* (1895), 496, cited by Horton-Smith, *op. cit.*, 1051.

21. A.S. Grünbaum, "The Goulstonian Lectures on Theories of Immunity and Their Clinical Application," *British Medical Journal* 1, no. 2204 (March 21, 1903): 653–655, 715–717.

22. "Obituary, Albert Sidney Frankau Leyton," *Lancet* 2, no. 5120 (October 15, 1921): 825–826.

23. A. Chantemesse and F. Widal, " De l'immunité contre le virus de la fièvre typhoïde conférée par des substances solubles," *Annales de l'institut Pasteur* 2 (1888): 54–59.

24. A. Chantemesse and F. Widal, *Annales de l'Institut Pasteur* (1892): 768, cited by P. Horton-Smith, "The Goulstonian Lectures on the Typhoid Bacillus and Typhoid Fever," *Lancet* 1, no. 3998 (April 14, 1900): 1050–1063.

25. Georges Dieulafoy, *A Text-book of Medicine*, vol. 2 (New York: D. Appleton, 1912), 1668.

26. Fernand Widal, "On the Sero-Diagnosis of Typhoid Fever," *Lancet* 2, no.

3820 (November 14, 1896): 1371–1372; Widal, *Bulletins et Mémoires de la Société des Hôpitaux de Paris* (June 26, 1896).

27. *New York Medical Journal* 48 (July 7, 1888) "Letter from Paris," 8. Drs. Oliver Wendell Holmes, father of the jurist, in Boston, and Ignaz Semmelweis in Vienna had demonstrated decades earlier that puerperal fever was often passed by physicians through unsanitary practices. The etiological agent was unknown at the time.

28. Albert Grünbaum, "Preliminary Note on the Use of the Agglutinative Action of Human Serum for the Diagnosis of Enteric Fever," *Lancet* 2, no. 3812 (September 19, 1896): 806–807.

29. Fernand Widal, "On the Sero-Diagnosis of Typhoid Fever," 1371–1372.

30. *Ibid.*

31. Grünbaum, *op. cit.*

Chapter 9

1. Robert Koch, "Die Bekämpfung des Typhus," *Veröffentlichungen aus dem Gebiete des Militär-Sanitätswesens* 21 (1903); August Hirschwald Verlag, Berlin ("The Control of Typhoid Fever," *Publications from the areas of Military*-Sanitation), cited in Thomas Brock, *Robert Koch: A Life in Medicine and Bacteriology* (Washington, DC: American Society for Microbiology, 1999), 256.

2. Arthur Blachstein, "Intravenous Inoculation of Rabbits with the Bacillus coli Communis and the Bacillus Typhi Abdominalis," *Johns Hopkins Hospital Bulletin* 14 (July 1891): 96–103.

3. William Welch, "Additional Note Concerning the Intravenous Inoculation of the Bacillus Typhi Abdominalis," *Johns Hopkins Hospital Bulletin* 15 (August 1891): 121–122.

4. William Park, "The Bacteriology of Typhoid Fever," *Medical News* 75 (December 16, 1899): 25–29.

5. *Ibid.*

6. P. Horton-Smith, "The Goulstonian Lectures on the Typhoid Bacillus and Typhoid Fever," *British Medical Journal* 1, no. 2049 (April 7, 1900): 827–834.

7. *Ibid.*, 828.

8. *Ibid.*, 830–831.

9. Brock, *op. cit.*, 255; http://www.learner.org/workshops/primarysources/disease/docs/park.html.

10. See citation 1.

11. J. Ledingham and J.A. Arkwright, *The Carrier Problem in Infectious Disease* (London: Edward Arnold, 1912), 6–7.

12. "Sources of Infection in Typhoid Fever," *Journal of the American Medical Association* 42, no. 24 (June 1, 1904): 1563.

13. Ledingham, *op. cit.*, 8–9.

14. *Ibid.*; Abraham Garbat, *Monographs of the Rockefeller Institute for Medical Research: Typhoid Carriers and Typhoid Immunity* (New York: Rockefeller Institute, 1922), 8.

15. William Park, "Typhoid Bacilli Carriers," *Journal of the American Medical Association* 51, no. 12 (September 19, 1908): 981.

16. Ledingham, *op. cit.*, 10.

17. Robert Crawford et al., "Gallstones Play a Significant Role in *Salmonella* spGallbladder Colonization and Carriage," *Proceedings National Academy of Sciences USA* 107, no. 9 (March 2, 2010): 4353–4358.

18. *Ibid.*

19. Judith Walzer Leavitt, *Typhoid Mary, Captive to the Public's Health* (Boston: Beacon Press, 1996), 14.

20. www.ancestry.com

21. George Soper, "The Work of a Chronic Typhoid Germ Distributor," *Journal of the American Medical Association* 48, no. 24 (June 15, 1907): 2019–2022.

22. George Soper, "The Curious Career of Typhoid Mary," *Bulletin of the New York Academy of Medicine* 15, no. 10 (1939): 698–712, cited by Leavitt, *op. cit.*, 170.

23. *Ibid.*, 699.

24. Soper, "Work of a Chronic Typhoid," *op. cit.*, 2022. Also cited by Leavitt, *op. cit.*, n4, 258. Also quoting from Leavitt (258–259): "I had read the address which Koch had delivered before the Kaiser Wilhelm's Akademic, November 28, 1902, and his investigation into the prevalence of typhoid at Trier, and thought it was one of the most illuminating of documents. In fact it had been the basis of much of the epidemic work with which I had been connected" (Soper). Exactly when Soper became aware of Koch's hypothesis of typhoid carriers is unclear. In his earlier investigations (c. 1904) he made no mention of possible carriers.

25. http://chroniclingamerica.loc.gov/lccn/sn83030214/1905-05-07/ed-1/seq-15/#date1=1890&index=1&rows=20&words=MRS+STRICKER&searchType=basic&sequence=0&state=New+York&date2=1910&proxtext=mrs.+stricker+&y=15&x=8&date

FilterType=yearRange&page=1. Mrs. Stricker's full name may have been Rosina Stricker, who was listed in the 1900 census as agency employer.

26. Soper, "Curious Career," *op. cit.*

27. According to records of the 1900 census, among the servants was Robert Lewis and his wife, Clara, Sarah Chenery, Delia Burns and Mary Barrett. Lewis, his wife and Sarah Chenery were born in Virginia. Since only Clara Lewis and Sarah Chenery fit the description of possible sisters—each born in Virginia—it is possible these were two of the victims, with Robert Lewis possibly a third. The gardener was a full time employee of the estate and was not a regular member of the household.

28. No indication of the name of the child could be found in either Soper's publications or the excellent biography of Mallon by Leavitt. New York City death records for the month of February 1907 yielded two possible names. Catherine Bowen, age 38, died on February 22, 1907. Since the only reference used by either Soper or Leavitt (likely Soper as the source) is that of a "lovely daughter," she would appear the likely victim. A second Bowen, Susan, aged 2 years, died February 4, 1907. The date would appear to rule her out.

29. Leavitt, *op. cit.*, 103.

30. Soper, "Curious Career," *op. cit.*, 698.

31. *Ibid.*, 704.

32. *Ibid.*, 704–705.

33. *Ibid.*, 705.

34. Hoobler, later head of Children's Hospital in Detroit, Michigan, was married late in life to Dr. Icie Macy Hoobler, a major figure during the 1930s on the subject of children's nutrition and growth. Her research at Children's Village in Redford, Michigan, focused on the relationship between diet and mother's milk.

35. Soper, "Curious Career," *op. cit.*

36. *Ibid.*, 706.

37. *Ibid.*

38. Park, "Typhoid Bacilli Carriers," *op. cit.*, 981.

39. Leavitt, *op. cit.*, 127.

40. Park, *op. cit.*, 982. In 1922 Rosenau helped establish the School of Public Health at Harvard University. In 1940, several years before his death, Rosenau was appointed as the first dean of the School of Public Health at the University of North Carolina.

41. Leavitt, *op. cit.*, 198.

42. Soper, "Curious Career," 712.

43. George Soper, "The Epidemic of Typhoid Fever at Ithaca, New York," *Journal of the New England Waterworks Association* 18, no. 4: 431–461.

44. *Ibid.*

45. George Soper, *The Air and Ventilation of Subways* (New York: John Wiley & Sons, 1908).

46. "Soper, Obituary," *New York Times*, June 18, 1948, p. 23.

47. http://www.gilderlehrman.org/history-by-era/essays/influenza-pandemic-1918%E2%80%931919; see also Richard Adler, *Victor Vaughan: A Biography of the Pioneering Bacteriologist* (Jefferson, NC: McFarland, 2015), 175–177.

Chapter 10

1. Michael Bliss, *William Osler: A Life in Medicine* (New York: Oxford University Press, 1999), 249.

2. Daniel Salmon, "Immunity from Contagious Diseases Produced by Products of Bacterial Multiplication," *Proceedings of the American Association for the Advancement of Science* 35 (August 1886): 258–262.

3. D.E. Salmon and T. Smith, "Report on Swine Plague," *U.S. Bureau of Animal Industries: 2nd Annual Report* (Washington, D.C.: U.S. Government Printing Office, 1885). The agent was often serendipitously referred to in publications as a virus, including the source quoted above, the term referring to a "poison" or infectious agent rather than the biological entity, as the term virus is recognized today. Of course, since it was later found to actually be a virus, the writers were correct for the wrong reason. See William Bulloch, *The History of Bacteriology* (New York: Dover, 1938), 256; Dieter Gröschel and Richard Hornick, "Who Introduced Typhoid Vaccination: Almroth Wright or Richard Pfeiffer?," *Reviews of Infectious Diseases* 3, no. 6 (November–December 1981): 1251–1254.

4. A. Wright, "On the Possible Advantages of Employing Decalcified Milk in the Feeding of Infants and Invalids," *Lancet* 2, no. 3647 (July 22, 1893): 194, and "Association of Serous Haemorrhages with Conditions of Defective Blood-Coagulability," *Lancet* 2, no. 3812 (September 19, 1896): 807–809.

5. *Ibid.*, 809.

6. *Op. cit.*, Gröschel.

7. W. Sirotinin, "Die Ubertragung von Typhusbacillen auf Versuchsthiere" [The Transmission of Typhoid Bacilli to Lower Animals] *Zeitschrift für Hygiene* 1 (May 1886): 465–488, cited by Gröschel.

8. E. Fraenkel and M. Simmonds, "Die Aetiologische Bedeutung des Typhus Bacillus" [The Etiological Significance of the Typhoid Bacillus] Hamburg/Leipzig, Voss, 1886; P.W. Latham et al., "The Pathology and Treatment of Typhoid Fever," *Lancet* 1, no. 3627 (March 4, 1893): 464–466, also cited by Gröschel.

9. Latham, *ibid.*; Joseph McFarland, *A Textbook upon the Pathogenic Bacteria* (Philadelphia: W.B. Saunders, 1903), 497.

10. E. Fraenkel, "Über specifische Behandlung des Abdominaltyphus" [About the Specific Treatment of Typhoid Fever], *Deutsche Med. Wochenschr* 19 (1893): 985–987, also cited by Gröschel.

11. R. Stern, "Über die Wirkung des menschlichen Blutserums auf die experimentelle Typhusinfection" [About the Effect of Human Blood Serum on Experimental Typhoid Infection] *Zeitschrift für Hygiene und Infektions Krankheiten* 16, no. 1 (1894): 458–481; Latham, *op. cit.*

12. Latham, *ibid.*

13. A.E. Wright and D. Semple, "Remarks on Vaccination Against Typhoid Fever," *British Medical Journal* 1, no. 1883 (January 30, 1897): 256–259; Michael Dunnill, *The Plato of Praed Street* (London: Royal Society of London Press, 2000), 54–55.

14. Ilana Lowy, "From Guinea Pigs to Man: The Development of Haffkine's Anticholera Vaccine," *Journal of the History of Medicine and Allied Sciences* 47 (1992): 270–309; Richard Adler, *Cholera in Detroit: A History* (Jefferson, NC: McFarland, 2013), 195–196.

15. Wright and Semple, *op. cit.*; also quoted by Gröschel, 1252.

16. A.E. Wright and D. Bruce, "On Haffkine's method of vaccination against Asiatic cholera," *British Medical Journal* 1, no. 1675 (February 4, 1893): 227–231; Barbara Hawgood, "Waldemar Mordecai Haffkine, CIE (1860–1930): Prophylactic Vaccination Against Cholera and Bubonic Plague in British India," *Journal of Medical Biography* 15 (2007): 9–19.

17. Hawgood, "Waldemar Mordecau Haffkine, CIE," 9–19.

18. Wright and Semple, "Remarks."

19. *Ibid.*

20. *Ibid.*

21. *Ibid.*

22. Wright and Semple, "Remarks"; Dunnill, *op. cit.*, 55.

23. Wright and Semple, "Remarks."

24. *Ibid.*

25. *Ibid.*

26. *Ibid.*

27. R. Pfeiffer and W. Kolle, "Experimentelle Untersuchungen zur Frage der Schutzimpfung des Menschen gegen Typhus abdominalis" [Experimental Studies to Test a Vaccine Against Typhoid in People], *Deutsche Medicinische Wochenschrift* 22, no. 46 (November 12, 1896): 735–737.

28. Wright and Semple, "Remarks."

29. Gröschel, *op. cit.*

30. A.E. Wright, *A Short Treatise on Antityphoid Inoculation* (Westminster, London: Archibald Constable, 1904), 19, quoted also by Gröschel.

31. Wright, *A Short Treatise*; Gröschel. It should be noted this interpretation by the authors (Mara and Adler) draws in part on the aforementioned published work by Gröschel and Hornick.

32. Gröschel, *op. cit.*

33. A.E. Wright and S.R. Stewart, "An Experimental Investigation of the Role of the Blood Fluids in Connection with Phagocytosis," *Proceedings of the Royal Society of London* 72 (1903): 357–370.

34. Wright and Semple, *op. cit.*

35. "Epidemic of Typhoid Fever at Maidstone," *British Medical Journal* 2, no. 1919 (October 9, 1897): 1022–1023; http://maidstonetyphoidepidemic.weebly.com/.

36. Christopher Collins, "Cholera and Typhoid Fever in Kent," Paper no. 4, www.kentarchaeology.ac (pp. 21–26).

37. Wright (1904) *op. cit.*, 53–54; Dunnill, *op. cit.*, 57.

38. Dunnill, 57–58.

39. A.E. Wright, "On the Results Which Have Been Obtained by the Anti-typhoid Inoculations," *Lancet* 1, no. 3986 (January 20, 1900): 150–153.

40. Dunnill, *op. cit.*, 58; "The Report of the Indian Plague Commission," *British Medical Journal* 1, no. 2157 (May 3, 1902): 1093–1098; also vol. 1, no. 2160 (May 24, 1902): 1279–1281.

41. Wright, "On the Results" (1900); Dunnill, 58.

42. Dunnill, 58–59.

43. Wright, "On the Results."

44. *Ibid.*

45. *Ibid.*

46. http://samilitaryhistory.org/vol063jc.html.

47. Dunnill, 61.

48. A.E. Wright, "A Note on the Results Obtained by the Anti-typhoid Inoculations in the Beleaguered Garrison in Ladysmith," *Lancet* 2, no. 4011 (July 14, 1900): 95.

49. Wright, *A Short Treatise*, 52–53.

50. Wright, "A Note on the Results" (1900).

51. Leonard Colebrook, "Obituary, Almroth Edward Wright," *Lancet* 1, no. 6454 (May 10, 1947): 654–656; Dunnill, 61.

52. Mazyck Ravenel, "The Control of Typhoid Fever by Vaccination," *Proceedings of the American Philosophical Society* 52, no. 209 (April 1913): 226–233.

53. Dunnill, *op. cit.*, 10–11. As related by Dunnill, Wooldridge was a prominent physiologist among whose achievements was the determination that the clotting of blood was not the property of the red blood cells but rather the result of processing of a protein in blood serum, fibrinogen, into fibrin. Among Wooldridge's students was Ernest Starling, later to become a major figure in the same field. Wooldridge died at the young age of 32, and his widow, Florence Wooldridge, subsequently married Starling. A colleague remarked, "I have heard of many reasons for getting married but never in order to get at the notebooks of your predecessor."

54. Colebrook, "Almroth Edward Wright." Roy, tragically, was a morphine addict who a decade later died during a fit. During his two years at Cambridge Wright transferred to the Department of Physiology, then under the chairmanship of Dr. Michael Foster (Dunnill, 12).

55. Dunnill, 13.

56. *Ibid.*, 19.

57. Colebrook, "Almroth Edward Wright," *Obituary Notices of the Royal Society* 6, no. 17, pp. 297–314.

58. *Ibid.*, 299. Numbers vary from "official" British statistics on the Boer War.

59. Abram Benenson, "Immunization and Military Medicine," *Reviews of Infectious Diseases* 6, no. 1 (January–February 1984): 1–12.

60. R. Germanier and E. Fürer, "Isolation and Characterization of *Gal* E Mutant Ty21a of *Salmonella typhi*: A Candidate Strain for a Live, Oral Typhoid Vaccine," *Journal of Infectious Diseases* 131, no. 5 (1975): 553–559.

61. A. Felix and R. Margaret Pitt, "A New Antigen of B. Typhosus: Its Relation to Virulence and to Active and Passive Immunisation," *Lancet* 224, no. 5787 (July 28, 1934): 186–191.

62. *Ibid.*

63. Iswar Acharya et al., "Prevention of Typhoid Fever with the Capsular Polysaccharide of *Salmonella typhi*," *New England Journal of Medicine* 317 (October 29, 1987): 1101–1106.

64. R. Schneerson et al., "Preparation, Characterization and Immunogenicity of *Haemophilus influenza* type b polysaccharide-protein conjugates," *Journal of Experimental Medicine* 152, no. 2 (August 1, 1980): 361–376.

65. Feng Ying Lin et al., "The Efficacy of a *Salmonella typhi* Vi Conjugate Vaccine in Two-To-Five-Year-Old Children," *New England Journal of Medicine* 344, no. 17 (April 26, 2001): 1263–1269.

Chapter 11

1. (Colonel) W.D. Tigertt, "The Initial Effort to Immunize American Soldier Volunteers with Typhoid Vaccine," *Military Medicine* 124, no. 5 (1959): 342–349.

2. Dwight Kuhns (M.D.) and (Capt.) Donald Learnard, "Typhoid and Paratyphoid Fevers," in *U.S. Army Medical Department, Office of Medical History*, chapter 22: 463.

3. *Medical and Surgical History of the War of the Rebellion*, Part 1, Vol. 1., *Medical History* (1870).

4. Drew Gilpin Faust, *This Republic of Suffering* (New York: Alfred A. Knopf, 2008), 4.

5. S.C. Gwynne, *Rebel Yell: The Violence, Passion, and Redemption of Stonewall Jackson* (New York: Scribner, 2014), 60.

6. Abram Benenson, "Immunization and Military Medicine," *Reviews of Infectious Diseases* 6, no. 1 (January–February 1984): 1–12.

7. Victor Vaughan, *A Doctor's Memories* (Indianapolis: Bobbs-Merrill, 1926), 370–371.

8. *Ibid.*, 372–373.

9. *Ibid.*, 371–372.

10. Bobby Wintermute, *Public Health and the US Military: A History of the Army Medical Department, 1818–1917* (New York: Routledge, 2011), 96.

11. Harry E. Webber, *Twelve Months with the Eighth Massachusetts Infantry in the Service of the United States* (Newcomb & Gauss, 1908), 87.

12. Richard Adler, *Victor Vaughan: The Biography of a Pioneering Bacteriologist* (Jefferson, NC: McFarland, 2014).

13. http://history.amedd.army.mil/books doc/wwii/PM4/CH22.Typhoid.htm.

14. Tigertt, 343.

15. *Ibid.*

16. In addition to Carroll, Vedder and Gilchrist, the ten volunteers were Sergeant Joseph Howe and Pvts. William Lumley, George Dunn, George Williams, George Ward, Robert Eisemann, Merl Clifford, William Epps, Claud Powell and Robert Bowman.

17. Tigertt, 344.

18. Benenson, 3.

19. Tigertt, 345–346.

20. *Ibid.*, 348.

21. *New York Times*, February 9, 1913, p. 8.

22. http://olive-drab.com/od_medical_other_lyster_bag.php.

23. http://history.amedd.army.mil/books doc/wwii/PM4/CH22.Typhoid.htm.

24. Arthur Gorman and Abel Wolman, *Water-borne Outbreaks in the United States and Canada and Their Significance* (New York: American Water Works Association, 1939), 40.

25. http://history.amedd.army.mil/books docs/wwii/PrsnlHlthMsrs/chapter8.htm.

26. *Ibid.*

27. Theodore Woodward et al., "Preliminary Report on the Beneficial Effect of Chloromycetin in the Treatment of Typhoid Fever," *Annals of Internal Medicine* 29, no. 1 (July 1, 1948): 131–134.

28. Theodore Woodward, Joseph Smadel and Herbert Levy, Jr., "Chloramphenicol and Other Antibiotics in the Treatment of Typhoid Fever and Typhoid Carriers," *Journal of Clinical Investigation* 29, no. 1 (January 1950): 87–99.

29. Thomas Timothy Crocker and Abraham Gelperin, "Treatment of the Typhoid Carrier State with Chloramphenicol," *Yale Journal of Biology and Medicine* 23, no. 2 (November 1950): 119–125.

30. http://usmilitary.about.com/od/the-orderlyroom/l/blvaccinations.htm.

31. www.vaccines.mil/documents/1593_SO_Typhoid_Fever_29_Nov_12.pdf.

Chapter 12

1. John Crump, "The Global Burden of Typhoid Fever," *Bulletin of the World Health Organization* 82, no. 5 (May 2004): 346–353.

2. Geoffrey Buckle, Christa L. Fischer Walker and Robert E. Black, "Typhoid Fever and Paratyphoid Fever: Systematic Review to Estimate Global Morbidity and Mortality for 2010," *Journal of Global Health* 2, no. 1 (June 2012); http://www.jogh.org/issue201201.htm.

3. *Ibid.*

4. Octavie Lunguya et al., "*Salmonella typhi* in the Democratic Republic of the Congo: Fluoroquinolone Decreased Susceptibility on the Rise," *PLoS Neglected Tropical Diseases* 6, no. 11 (November 2012): e1921.

5. K.H. Keddy et al., "Molecular Epidemiological Investigation of a Typhoid Fever Outbreak in Delmas, South Africa, 2005: The Relationship to a Prior Epidemic in 1993," *Epidemiology and Infection* 139 (2011): 1239–1245.

6. Buckle, *op. cit.*

7. Gardiner Harris, "'Superbugs' Kill India's Babies and Pose an Overseas Threat," *New York Times*, December 4, 2014, p. A1.

8. "Typhoid Fever Surveillance and Vaccine Use: South-East Asia and Western Pacific Regions, 2009–2013," *Morbidity and Mortality Weekly Report* 63, no. 39 (October 3, 2014): 855–860.

9. *Morbidity and Mortality Weekly Report* 51, no. 53 (April 30, 2004): 13.

10. Stephen Berger, *Infectious Diseases of the United States, 2013*, 1119 pages, 470 graphs, 11030 references. Gideon e-books, http://www.gideononline.com/ebooks/coun try/infectious-diseases-of-the-united-states.

11. Kamaljit Singh, "Laboratory-Acquired Infections," *Clinical Infectious Diseases* 49, no. 1 (July 1, 2009): 142–147.

12. David Sewell, "Laboratory-Associated Infections and Biosafety," *Clinical Microbiology Reviews* 8, no. 3 (July 1995): 389–405.

13. Bradley Conner and Eli Schwartz, "Typhoid and Paratyphoid Fever in Travelers," *Lancet Infectious Diseases* 5 (2005): 623–628.

14. *Ibid.*

Bibliography

Books

Adler, Richard. *Cholera in Detroit: A History.* Jefferson, NC: McFarland, 2013.
_____. *Victor Vaughan: A Biography of the Pioneering Bacteriologist.* Jefferson, NC: McFarland, 2015.
Allen, Arthur. *The Fantastic Laboratory of Dr. Weigl.* New York: W.W. Norton, 2014.
Ashwal, Stephen. "William Gerhard," in *The Founders of Child Neurology.* Edited by Stephen Ashwal (San Francisco: Norman, 1990), 122.
Bartlett, Elisha. *The History, Diagnosis and Treatment of Typhoid and of Typhus Fever.* Philadelphia: Lea and Blanchard, 1842.
Bauer, K. Jack. *Zachary Taylor: Soldier, Planter, Statesman of the Old Southwest.* Baton Rouge: Louisiana State University Press, 1985.
Bliss, Michael. *William Osler: A Life in Medicine.* New York: Oxford University Press, 1999.
Bolduan, Charles Frederick, and John Koopman. *Immune Sera: A Concise Exposition of our Present Knowledge of Infection and Immunity.* New York: John Wiley & Sons, 1917.
Brock, Thomas. *Robert Koch: A Life in Medicine and Bacteriology.* Washington, D.C.: American Society for Microbiology, 1999.
Budd, William. *On the Causes of Fevers* (1839). Edited by Dale. Baltimore, MD: Johns Hopkins University Press, 1984.
_____. *Typhoid Fever: Its Nature, Mode of Spreading, and Prevention.* London: Longmans, Green, 1873.
Bulloch, William. *The History of Bacteriology.* New York: Dover, 1938.
Bynum, W.F., and Roy Porter, ed. *Companion Encyclopedia of the History of Medicine.* London: Routledge, 1993.
Chinnock, E.J. *The Anabasis of Alexander; or, The History of the Wars and Conquests of Alexander the Great.* "Literally Translated, with a Commentary, from the Greek of Arrian the Nicomedian." London: Hodder and Stoughton, 1884.
Chugg, Andrew. *The Quest for the Tomb of Alexander the Great.* AMC, 2007.
Coulter, Harris L. *Divided Legacy: A History of the Schism in Medical Thought.* Berkeley, CA: North Atlantic Books, 2000.
Curschmann, H. *Typhoid Fever and Typhus Fever.* Edited by William Osler. Philadelphia: W.B. Saunders, 1901.
de Hildenbrand, Johann Valentin. Translated by S.D. Gross. *A Treatise on the Nature, Cause, and Treatment of Contagious Typhus.* New York: Elam Bliss, 1829.
Dieulafoy, Georges. *A Text-book of Medicine.* Vol. 2. New York: D. Appleton, 1912.

Dixon, Karen, and Pat Southern. *The Roman Cavalry.* New York: Routledge, 1997.

Dorfman, Robert, Henry Jacoby and Harold Thomas. *Models for Managing Regional Water Quality.* Cambridge, MA: Harvard University Press, 1972.

Dubos, René. *Louis Pasteur: Free Lance of Science.* New York: Da Capo, 1960.

Dunnill, Michael. *The Plato of Praed Street.* London: Royal Society of London Press, 2000.

Encyclopedia of Microbiology. 2nd ed. New York: Academic Press, 2000.

Faust, Drew Gilpin. *This Republic of Suffering.* New York: Alfred A. Knopf, 2008.

"Febris Gallica, epidemia." In *Bibliotheca Medico-Practica.* Geneva: Haeredum Cramer & Fratrum Philibert, 1739.

Garbat, Abraham. *Monographs of the Rockefeller Institute for Medical Research: Typhoid Carriers and Typhoid Immunity.* New York: Rockefeller Institute, 1922.

Garrison, Fielding H. *An Introduction to the History of Medicine.* Philadelphia: W.B. Saunders, 1922.

Gay, Frederick Parker. *Typhoid Fever Considered as a Problem of Scientific Medicine.* New York: Macmillan, 1918.

Geison, Gerald. *The Private Science of Louis Pasteur.* Princeton, NJ: Princeton University Press, 1995.

Gill, Gillian. *We Two: Victoria and Albert, Rulers, Partners, Rivals.* Ballantine Books, 2009.

Gorman, Arthur, and Abel Wolman. *Water-borne Outbreaks in the United States and Canada and Their Significance.* New York: American Water Works Association, 1939.

Grove, David L. *Tapeworms, Lice and Prions: A Compendium of Unpleasant Infections.* New York: Oxford University Press, 2014.

Gwynne, S.C. *Rebel Yell: The Violence, Passion, and Redemption of Stonewall Jackson.* New York: Scribner, 2014.

Herodotus. *The Histories.* Translated by George Rawlinson. digireads.com publishing, 2009.

Hibbert, Christopher. *Queen Victoria: A Personal History.* Cambridge, MA: Da Capo, 2001.

Hippocrates. *The Genuine Works of Hippocrates.* Vol. 1. Translated from the Greek by Francis Adams, LLD. London: Sydenham Society, 1849.

Hudson, Alfred. *Lectures on the Study of Fever.* Philadelphia: Henry C. Lea, 1869.

Jenner, William. *On the Identity or Non-Identity of the Specific Cause of Typhoid, Typhus and Relapsing Fever.* London: John Churchill, 1850.

Leavitt, Judith Walzer. *Typhoid Mary: Captive to the Public's Health.* Boston: Beacon Press, 1996.

Ledingham, J., and J.A Arkwright. *The Carrier Problem in Infectious Disease.* London: Edward Arnold, 1912.

Mackowiak, Philip A. *Post Mortem.* Philadelphia: American College of Physicians, 2007.

Major, Ralph, ed. *Classic Descriptions of Disease.* IL: Charles C. Thomas, 1945.

Mazumdar, Pauline. *Species and Specificity.* New York: Cambridge University Press, 1995.

McCullough, David. *The Greater Journey: Americans in Paris.* New York: Simon & Schuster, 2011.

McFarland, Joseph. *A Textbook Upon the Pathogenic Bacteria.* Philadelphia: W.B. Saunders, 1903.

Murchison, Charles. *A Treatise on the Continued Fevers of Great Britain.* 3rd ed. London: Longmans, Green, 1884.

Osler, W. *The Principles and Practice of Medicine.* 8th ed. London: Appleton, 1919.

Plutarch. *Lives.* Vol. 7. Cambridge, MA: Harvard University Press, 1958.

Porter, Roy. *The Greatest Benefit to Mankind: A Medical History of Humanity.* New York: W.W. Norton, 1997.

Raoult, D., and M. Drancourt, ed. *Paleomicrobiology: Past Human Infections.* Berlin: Springer-Verlag, 2008.

Ridley, Jane. *The Heir Apparent: A Life of Edward VII, the Playboy Prince.* New York: Random House, 2014.

Roger, Henri. *Infectious Diseases: Their Etiology, Diagnosis and Treatment.* New York: Lea Brothers, 1903.

Salmon, D.E., and T. Smith. "Report on Swine Plague." *U.S. Bureau of Animal Industries, 2nd Annual Report.* Washington, D.C.: U.S. Government Printing Office, 1885.

Scarry, Robert J. *Millard Fillmore.* Jefferson, NC: McFarland, 2001.

Schaechter, Moselio, ed.-in-chief. *Encyclopedia of Microbiology.* San Diego: Elsevier/Academic, 2009.

Simmons, John G. *Doctors and Discoveries: Lives That Created Today's Medicine.* Boston, MA: Houghton Mifflin, 2002.

Smith, Theobald. *Special Report on the Cause and Prevention of Swine Plague.* Washington, D.C.: Government Printing Office, 1891.

Soper, George. *The Air and Ventilation of Subways.* New York: John Wiley & Sons, 1908.

Southern, Patricia. *Augustus.* 2nd ed. New York: Routledge, 2014.

Suetonius. *The Twelve Caesars.* Book II. *Augustus,* LIX. "Offerings and Commemorations." A.S Kline (Translation), 2010.

Thayer, Bill. *The Library of History of Diodorus Siculus.* Loeb Classic Library Edition. Vol. 8, Book 17. 1963.

Vaughan, Victor. *A Doctor's Memories.* Indianapolis: Bobbs-Merrill, 1926.

Vaughan, Victor C., Henry F. Vaughan and George T. Palmer. *Epidemiology and Public Health.* Vol. II. St. Louis: C.V. Mosby, 1923.

Webber, Harry E. *Twelve Months with the Eighth Massachusetts Infantry in the Service of the United States.* Newcomb & Gauss, 1908.

Weintraub, Stanley. *Victoria.* New York: E.P. Dutton, 1988.

Welch, William Henry. *Papers and Addresses by William Henry Welch.* Vol. 1. Baltimore: Johns Hopkins University Press, 1920.

_____. *Papers and Addresses.* Vol. 2, *Bacteriology.* Baltimore: Johns Hopkins University Press, 1920.

Whipple, George Chandler. *Typhoid Fever: Its Causation, Transmission and Prevention.* New York: John Wiley & Sons, 1908.

Wintermute, Bobby. *Public Health and the US Military: A History of the Army Medical Department, 1818–1917.* New York: Routledge, 2011.

Wright, A.E. *A Short Treatise on Anti-typhoid Inoculation.* Westminster, London: Archibald Constable, 1904.

Periodicals

American Farmer: A Monthly Magazine of Agriculture and Horticulture
American Journal of Epidemiology
American Journal of Medicine
American Journal of the Medical Sciences
Annales de l'Institut Pasteur
Annals of Internal Medicine
Annals of Microbiology
Boston Medical and Surgical Journal
British Medical Journal
Bulletin of the New York Academy of Medicine
Bulletin of the Society of Medical History of Chicago
Bulletin of the World Health Organization
Bulletins et Mémoires de la Société des Hôpitaux de Paris
Cell Host and Microbe

Cellular Immunology
Cellular Microbiology
Classical Quarterly
Clinical Infectious Diseases
Clinical Microbiology Reviews
Deutsche medicinische Wochenschrift
Dublin Journal of Medical Science
Edinburgh Monthly Journal of Medical Medicine
Epidemiology and Infection
Epidemiology and Public Health
Infection and Immunity
Infectious Disease Clinics of North America
Johns Hopkins Hospital Bulletin
Journal of Clinical Investigation
Journal of Clinical Microbiology
Journal of Experimental Medicine
Journal of Global Health
Journal of Infectious Diseases
Journal of Laboratory and Clinical Medicine
Journal of Medical Biography
Journal of Physiology and Pharmacology
Journal of the American Medical Association
Journal of the History of Medicine
Journal of the History of Medicine and Allied Sciences
Journal of the New England Waterworks Association
Journal of the Royal Society of Medicine
Lancet
Lancet Infectious Diseases
London Medical and Surgical Journal
London Medical Repository, Monthly Journal and Review
London Observer
Medical and Surgical History of the War of the Rebellion
Medical Communications of the Massachusetts Medical Society
Medical History
Medical News
Medico-Chirurgical Transactions
Microbes and Infection
Microbiological Research
Military Medicine
Morbidity and Mortality Weekly Report
Münchener medicinische Wochenschrift
Nature
New England Journal of Medicine
New York Medical Journal
New York Times
Obituary Notices of the Royal Society
Paleomicrobiology: Past Human Infections
PLoS Neglected Tropical Diseases
Plumbers Trade Journal
Polish Journal of Pathology
Proceedings of the American Association for the Advancement of Science
Proceedings of the American Philosophical Society

Proceedings of the National Academy of Sciences USA
Proceedings of the Royal Society
Public Health Reports
Reviews of Infectious Diseases
Southeast Asian Journal of Tropical Medicine and Public Health
Transactions of the Royal Medical and Chirurgical Society
U.S. Bureau of Animal Industries: 2nd Annual Report
Washington Post
Wiener Klinische Wochenschrift
Yale Journal of Biology and Medicine
Zeitschrift für Hygiene
Zeitschrift für Hygiene und Infektions Krankheiten

Websites

Ackerknecht, Erwin Heinz. *Medicine at the Paris Hospital, 1794–1848.* Baltimore: Johns Hopkins Press, 1967. www.mini4stroke.tweakdsl.nl/Histmedsc/Ackerknecht.pdf.
Ancestry.com. http://www.ancestry.com.
Berger, Stephen. "Infectious Diseases of the United States." Gideon Ebooks, 2015. http://www.gideononline.com/ebooks/country/infectious-diseases-of-the-united-states.
Buckle, Geoffrey C., Christa L. Fischer-Walker, and Robert E. Black (2012). "Typhoid Fever and Paratyphoid Fever: Systematic Review to Estimate Global Morbidity and Mortality for 2010." *Journal of Global Health*, 2 (1). http://www.jogh.org/doc uments/issue201201/9-Article%20Buckle.pdf.
Byerly, Carol. "The Influenza Pandemic of 1918–1919." *History Now 40*, 2014. http:// www.gilderlehrman.org/history-by-era/essays/influenza-pandemic-1918%E2%80 %931919.
"Death of Alexander." http://hellenspot.narod.ru/page3.htm.
de Villiers, J.C. "The Medical Aspect of the Anglo-Boer War." *Military History Journal* 6 (3). A publication of the South African Military History Society, 1984. http:// samilitaryhistory.org/vol063jc.html.
"Durham, Herbert Edward." Catalog entry from London School of Hygiene and Tropical Medicine. http://www.aim25.ac.uk/cats/37/8112.htm.
Enersen, Ole Daniel. "Thomas Willis." Whonamedit.com. http://www.whonamedit. com/doctor.cfm/336.html.
Glass, Andrew. "Zachary Taylor's Body Exhumed, June 17, 1991." Politico.com, 2011. http://www.politico.com/news/stories/0611/57126.html.
Jones, W.H.S., ed. "Greek Medicine and Hippocrates." In *Hippocrates Collected Works I.* Cambridge: Harvard University Press, 1868. Accessed through Perseus Digital Library: http://www.perseus.tufts.edu/hopper/text?doc=Perseus:text:1999.01.0251: text=intro.
Kent Archaeological Society. www.kentarchaeology.ac.
"Koch, Heinrich Hermann Robert." Encyclopedia.com. http://www.encyclopedia.com/ topic/Robert_Koch.aspx.
Kohn, George Childs. "French Army Syphilis Epidemic." *Encyclopedia of Plague and Pestilence, Third Edition.* New York: Facts on File, 2007. *Modern World History Online.* http://www.fofweb.com/History/MainPrintPage.asp?iPin=ENPP205& DataType=WorldHistory.
Kuhns, Dwight M., and Donald L. Learnard. "Chapter XXII: Typhoid and Paratyphoid Fevers." In *Preventive Medicine in WWII, Volume IV, Communicable Diseases, Transmitted Chiefly Through Respiratory and Alimentary Tracts.* Washington, D.C.:

Department of the Army, 1958. http://history.amedd.army.mil/booksdocs/wwii/PM4/CH22.Typhoid.htm.

"Lyster Bag." Olive-drab.com. http://olive-drab.com/od_medical_other_lyster_bag.php.

"The Maidstone Typhoid Epidemic, 1897–1898." http://maidstonetyphoidepidemic.weebly.com/.

"Military Vaccinations." USmilitary.about.com. http://usmilitary.about.com/od/theorderlyroom/l/blvaccinations.htm.

"Mrs. R. Stricker and Nephew." Advertisement in *The New York Daily Tribune*, May 7, 1905. http://chroniclingamerica.loc.gov/lccn/sn83030214/1905-05-07/ed-1/seq-15/#date1=1890&index=1&rows=20&words=MRS+STRICKER&searchType=basic&sequence=0&state=New+York&date2=1910&proxtext=mrs.+stricker+&y=15&x=8&dateFilterType=yearRange&page=1.

Oak Ridge National Laboratory, http://web.ornl.gov/info/ornlreview/rev27-12/text/ansside6.html.

Park, William H. "Typhoid Bacilli Carriers." Primary Sources: Workshops in American History, http://www.learner.org/workshops/primarysources/disease/docs/park.html.

Siculus, Diodorus. "Library of History." Trans. C. Bradford Welles. In *Loeb Classical Library*, Vol. 8. Harvard University Press, 1963. http://penelope.uchicago.edu/Thayer/E/Roman/Texts/Diodorus_Siculus/17F*.html.

Seybert, Tony. "The Strange Death of Zachary Taylor." Daily Kos. http://www.dailykos.com/story/2005/05/29/117856/-THE-STRANGE-DEATH-OF-ZACHARY-TAYLOR#.

Suetonius. "Book II: Augustus." Trans. A. S. Kline. In *The Twelve Caesars*. Poetry in Translation, 2010. http://www.poetryintranslation.com/PITBR/Latin/Suetonius2.htm#_Toc276121921.

Thucydides. *The History of the Peloponnesian War*. Book II. Trans. Richard Crawley, http://classics.mit.edu/Thucydides/pelopwar.2.second.html.

Index

Numbers in **bold italics** indicate pages with photographs.